T0132450

# The Role of Exercise in Anti Aging

Dr. Goh Kong Chuan

iUniverse, Inc.
New York   Bloomington

iUniverse books may be ordered through booksellers or by contacting:

iUniverse
1663 Liberty Drive
Bloomington, IN 47403
www.iuniverse.com
1-800-Authors (1-800-288-4677)

ISBN: 978-1-4401-8487-1 (sc)
ISBN: 978-1-4401-8486-4 (ebook)

Printed in the United States of America

iUniverse rev. date: 12/17/2009

# Contents

# Foreword

In this 21$^{st}$ century, one is more conscious of the importance of maintaining one's health and youthfulness. Good health is not just a matter of genes or fate. Something else can be done about it. Exercise is universally recognized as an important way of maintaining good health. There is a profusion of fitness or wellness centers recommending various types of exercise. But commercialism is also playing a big part in the effort to maintain youthful looks. Everyday, we are bombarded with advertisements enticing people to maintain a youthful face and figure through dieting, pills, injections and even cosmetic and replacement surgery. All this is aimed at people in their middle years.

However, Dr. Goh Kong Chuan is one of the few who is in the forefront of the effort to help people maintain good health through exercise not just when young and during middle age, but also in old age. As a specialist in Sports Medicine, he is, of course, concerned with injuries sustained through sporting activities, but more importantly, he is concerned with the maintenance of good health into old age and has made this his passion and quest. He has found that it is the discipline of keeping to a regime of systematic and regular exercise that is the key to ensuring good health.

During the middle years, career and family commitments do take precedence, and the week-end warrior can only find time for the occasional hike up the hill, a swim, or occasional golf, badminton, tennis, or any other game that is enjoyable. But, it is never too late, even in retirement, for Dr. Goh constantly urges everyone to incorporate regular exercise into their daily regime to attain good health, as this is the only way to guarantee good quality of life and an active old age.

I am one who is fortunate and privileged to have the constant advice and encouragement from Dr. Goh to maintain a regime of regular exercise. Upon reaching the 70s and 80s, we inevitably suffer the aches and pains of old age, but in my personal experience, I have managed to minimize them through Dr. Goh's advice and encouragement with regular exercise.

I am now 88 years old, and have been suffering from bad Arthritis in both knees for more than 20 years, but through regular exercise I have been able to avoid medication or surgery, and am still able to enjoy a comfortable life. I can still engage in reasonably active holidays with my grand children and great grand children.

I unconditionally endorse Dr. Goh's message that one need not be worried about an uncomfortable or painful old age. There is certainly no need to have visions of being confined to a rocking chair or a wheelchair. For all this I have to thank Dr. Goh Kong Chuan.

By Nelly Lim (Oh)

# Dedication

This book is dedicated to my children and grandchildren to whom I want to pass this message so that they may enjoy Quality Life.

# Acknowledgement

To my loving wife, Florence who has been my constant companion and guide through this long journey. She has been my source of inspiration and encouragement, and all I have achieved is due to her.

# 1
# INTRODUCTION

When you reach the senior age of 65, you get the concessions that senior citizens are given  It also comes with the infirmities of aging, and I hope that this book will encourage you to enjoy quality life as some of us do. It will discuss how exercise can help us, and the popular modes of exercise that I have gone through as a doctor, a participant, and as one who has trained many in these same modes of exercise.

As a Sports Medicine Doctor, I work not with the elite athletes, but the majority of average exercisers who seek only to *exercise for health*. Everybody gives this stock answer when asked if he is really serious about his exercise, but do they all exhibit good health without the need for any medicine or supplement? If so, then they have indeed found the perfect exercise, and we can all learn from them. Unfortunately this is not always the case. I can show by personal example that this is possible if we exercise enough, and I will tell you how to go about it as you read on.

All of us need to exercise more, and if we can do so without suffering from the pitfalls of exercise, then we can really enjoy the benefits it will bring. I have gone through it, and continue to exercise many times a day. This book is an account of my experience, and will give you an idea of what is available out there. You will not find many references because these are mostly observations I have made from my experience, and classified as "anecdotal". What the establishment and popular media promote is not producing the results it promises, and it is time to act on our own observations, but we do not encourage you to stop your medication that may be necessary to treat your present illness.

Health trends change with the fashions and there is something basically wrong when so much ill health comes from following what is popular. I urge you to look at it objectively and follow what works. Just make a start, and don't be only a spectator, watching from a chair; we have turned into a generation of spectators who are good at reeling off names of the famous sportsmen who excel at their sports. We can only become healthy if we ourselves do something instead of imagining that we are the champions out there winning the medals.

By nature we are all competitive and we can fuel this competitiveness and harness it as the motivation we need to continue exercise by competing in endurance events that I indulge in many times a day. (I came out World #2 in open age group competition in endurance rowing at the age of 67 last October).

I have treated many elderly patients who really demonstrate anti aging by showing me the medals they have won after rehabilitating from injuries, surgery and other degenerative diseases through properly guided exercise.

This is some of the experience I will share with you in this book.

The topic of anti aging brings to mind many academic issues, the bottom line being how much money this fashionable idea will bring in. We need to be practical, instead of just talking until the cows come home, and imagining ourselves to be as young as we once were. Many new ideas will be presented and hopefully this will stimulate some paradigm shifts in thinking and behavior that will bring about changes.

There are many anti aging measures, but this book will concentrate on exercise, consistency in practice and faithful recording of your daily exercise workout. Exercise is one of the most cost-effective ways to achieve long-lasting results. Exercise helps to keep us young and healthy. This is often taken for granted, and people only pay lip service when they compliment the elderly who have managed to "look younger than their years". It is only when we approach the senior age of 65 that we become conscious of anti aging. The youngster never dreams that it will happen to him some day, and only wants to enjoy life and take whatever comes as fated, or as they say, *Kismet* (in the old romantic movie of years gone by). We are only mortal, and as we all inevitably age, we seek to regain what we have lost, and try to preserve whatever we have left in this quest for anti aging. There is no way to stop the aging process, and we seek only to slow it down and "Add (Quality) Life to our Years" and not just "Years to our Life".

Nowadays it is fashionable to pay for services and flaunt your wealth so that most people think they can buy their health, and not work for it. This leads to the focus on buying supplements and all sorts of beauty aids to make us "look and feel young". Anti aging Medicine has been commercially and cosmetically driven. So an industry flourishes, as the old generally have accumulated more wealth than the youngsters who have so many obligations early in their life. The rich may count all their worldly possessions, but they cannot carry it with them when eventually they have to go to meet their maker. We should try to "Add Life to our Years", and not just seek to add "Years to our Life" because it is only our maker who can do so. If we can function as well as we did when we were once young, that is more important than just looking young or feeling that we are young.

This is a book written to tell you that we can all achieve quality life if we work for it, even as we age. No man-made product can copy the body's own natural ability to preserve itself, and the secret is to learn how to make our bodies react to this natural tendency they have of rejuvenation. All the exercises described in this book have been tested out, and can be performed by perfectly normal people. All throughout, the emphasis is on using simple exercise to give us quality life as we all age, and to cut down our medical bills and doctor visits. There is no point in sounding very clever at dinner conversations about the latest diet or lifestyle changes, but never put it into practice consistently. What is the point of having a superb blood sugar level or extremely low bad cholesterol when you are taking tons of pills every morning, and hardly able to walk unaided? Some people may fool themselves that they are doing the right thing, but what sort of quality life do they lead in a wheel chair when their contemporaries are prancing around touring all the exotic places?

There are so many modes of exercise, and everyone feels that he is practicing the best that his experience has taught him. So let us try to discover these little "secrets" the seniors have to teach us. Variety may be the spice of life, but must we impose it so strictly when we have found one mode of exercise that really suits us and that we enjoy? There may seem to be emphasis on one mode of exercise that I have found most valuable, but the choice is yours, and the reader is exposed to most of the popular modes of exercise without having to go out to try them, and learn the hard way from his own mistakes. That is the purpose of reading- to tap the experience of someone who has gone through it himself.

My mission is to impress upon everyone the value of exercise, because all the old Sages and Hermits have shown us that they have achieved Quality Life through the discipline of meditation, seclusion and exercise they have cultivated. But we can mix this discipline with the enjoyable social life we need as human beings.

## Aerobic Exercise

Aerobic exercise is the cornerstone of quality life, as it trains up our cardiovascular system (heart and lungs) to withstand the needs of moving around, and we need to do so to distinguish us from the stationary trees that stay rooted to one spot forever. Then, of course, we have to develop our muscles to enable us to move around without feeling any pain or weakness.

There you have it- the ultimate "Secret of the seniors"- to move around freely without pain or weakness. But, of course, the mind must be clear and agile, to enjoy what we see (or hear) when we move around.

## The Gym

The newcomer to the gym is faced with a bewildering choice of modes of exercise, and every respectable gym will show off its status symbols:

- the most expensive treadmills (like the $30,000 HP Cosmo),
- the most fashionable cross trainers
- the latest single-station weight training machines, etc.

The newcomer gets so confused that he meekly looks at the regular gym users, and follows what they do. This is not the best way to go about it, and in the following chapters we will give you an idea of what each machine (or the outdoors) does for you.

It is like shopping for the best medicine for your ailment. In the case of an illness, you can trust your Doctor, but for exercise, should you trust the personal trainer or the physiotherapist, or the well meaning know-it-all who talks the most at dinner conversations and in the gyms? There are Doctors trained in Sports Medicine, Exercise Physiology, and Rehabilitation Medicine, and these should be the experts you should look to for advice on any aspect of exercise because they can read (with full understanding and interpretation) the latest journals and recommendations on exercise written up by the experts in the field.

After all, you don't take the medicine your friend takes, or the cheapest one you can buy at the drug store. Everyone is smart enough to know that a proper examination and diagnosis should be sought before taking the medicine best suited for the illness so diagnosed by the doctor. In the same way, you should choose the best mode of exercise for your goals. It might be simply to get fit, or to lose weight, or to strengthen your back that has been giving a nagging pain, or to rehabilitate from some injury.

Bearing in mind these goals, how do we achieve them- that is what I will attempt to tell you in this book.

## Key points

- Exercise is the most cost-effective way to achieve long-lasting anti aging
- We cannot stop the aging process, but can "Add (Quality) Life to your Years".
- We can achieve quality life by exercising towards it and recording it
- Aerobic exercise- the cornerstone of quality life
- Regard exercise as a prescription

# 2
# The Indoor Rower

This is the most under-utilized machine in most gyms, but gives the best all-round exercise. Compared to all other modes of exercise, this uses most of the muscles and joints of the body, and there are many free sites on the web where diagrams of the muscles used during the various stages of rowing are detailed. One of these is the home site of one of the manufacturers, Concept2, and can easily be found on the web.

Basically, it spares the knees, but builds up the bones and muscles, and gives the best cardiovascular exercise.[i] This is ideal for those who suffer from Osteoarthritis of the knees, and believe they can no longer exercise. Those who give up exercise totally because of this excuse become fat and show their age soon, and the inevitable signs of aging are upon them before they realize it. Our older cover girl has been suffering from Osteoarthritis of both knees, but instead of giving up exercise when she could not walk far, she took up Indoor Rowing, and has remained healthy even at the age of 88. The author himself would have been sidelined with Achilles Tendinosis if he had followed the advice of well-meaning healthcare professionals.

In Osteoporosis, the alternate compression and distraction of the bone stimulate the bone to grow, and this was first highlighted by the Veterinary Surgeon, Lanyon in the ACSM Position Stand on Osteoporosis in the late 1990s, and in the article by Andrew Hamilton BSc Hons MRSC [ii].

In this article he highlights the value of Indoor Rowing in *building up the bones* while *taking the stress off the knee*. This is the essence of this particular mode of exercise- Indoor Rowing, as it benefits those suffering from Osteoporosis and Osteoarthrits - the two commonest ailments that afflict most people, and on whom millions of $ are spent each year seeking cures. There are many such examples, but it will take too long to recount all of them, though we have attempted to illustrate this with some examples in Chapter 9 on Rehabilitation.

The Concept2 Indoor Rower is a simple machine that evolved from an overturned bicycle the two Dreissigacker brothers worked on when they were training at on-water rowing They found that the rivers were frozen in winter, but they still managed to train indoors for the whole year on this machine that they had invented. Eventually one of them represented the US at the Munich Olympics, and the Concept2 Indoor Rower has since been accepted as the training tool by all Olympians. There are now Indoor Rowing races organized in many countries throughout the World, and the UK has introduced its use in the schools recently.

To use the Indoor Rower, sit down on the machine, pushing your legs forward while pulling on the handle, which moves an accurately calibrated flywheel through the rower's chain. The display monitor has been cleverly designed to display Calories, Pace, Watts, Heart Rate, and even a pace boat function, while a smart log card records all your workouts automatically, taking the effort out of doing this manually.

This is a machine that lets you accurately record every facet of your workout, and train at any intensity you feel comfortable at. All the muscles of the body are worked, when you lean forwards and backwards, pushing with your legs and pulling in towards your midriff. Flexibility is also taken care of, and Osteoporosis is tackled as the bones get alternately compressed and distracted. This distortion of the bone beyond the Minimum Effective Strain (MES) stimulates the bone to grow, and was the principle Lanyon followed when he worked on animals to show that he could stimulate bone growth in them. It was in fact stated in the ACSM Position stand on Osteoporosis in the 1990s. NASA astronauts under the care of the famous middle distance runner at the Tokyo Olympics Dr. Peter Snell in Dallas now use the Indoor Rower to prevent the Osteoporosis they suffer from when weightless for long periods in space. Previously they had tried all sorts of gym equipment in their space capsule, and still came down with Osteoporosis. Most of the muscles of the body are used in the rowing stroke, and we realize that this is the complete exercise when we start Indoor Rowing. Besides the muscles used, flexibility of the joints is achieved with every stroke, and the slow powerful rhythmic strokes pose no danger to the body, while developing the heart slowly.

Many Dragon Boat Rowers and Kayakers have the misconception that they are automatically good at the sport of Indoor Rowing (without having to learn even the very basics), but none has managed to win at this Olympic Sport. Rowing has been established as one of the glamour sports in the Olympics, and Indoor Rowing is always taught before the Rowing Instructor lets you go out on water in the rowing shell. Indoor Rowing is a fluid motion that concentrates more on the legs than the arms, and this lesson must be drummed in to all who have the misconception that it only involves the upper body. You need a qualified Indoor Rowing instructor to show you how to do it properly without suffering from the injuries that many complain of.

There is also the wrong concept that the resistance must be pushed to the maximum at "10", with all the air vents open. This is like driving a car at 1st gear, and redlining it while going up to a maximum speed of 60kph. The guy who rows with a damper setting of "3" is like one who drives the car on 4th gear, and can fly along silently at 250 Km/h. World champion rowers like Rob Waddell are 6'9.5" tall, and weigh 230 lbs, and yet they keep the damper setting at "3". So there is no need for the average rower who may be only 5'9" and weighing 160lb to put his damper setting at "10". (*The empty vessel makes the most noise*).

Personal trainers, rehabilitation professionals and cardiac rehabilitation specialists should learn how to row and add this piece of machinery to their arsenal instead of sticking to their conventional equipment and criticizing the Indoor Rower that is producing amazing results in rehabilitation. My website has recorded the heart rate of a heart bypass (CABG) patient spiking many times above 220bpm when walking slowly on the treadmill, while recording a steady 115 beats per minute when seated and rowing hard for >1 hour. This can be found at http://wwwoarobics-malaysia.com, and seen in Fig.1 below. There are also many reports of the elderly suffering from fractures, Osteoporosis, Osteoarthritis or just after Surgery who have rehabilitated (on the Indoor Rower) in record time to win Gold medals in exhausting competition and returned to show their achievements. This will be covered in Chapter 9 when we talk about Rehabilitation.

So many Heart Bypass patients have rowed their way to health, without even a single cardiac event, and even a Heart Transplant patient and many with Implanted Defibrillators have used it. See the chart below that shows a comparison of a Heart Bypass Patient while walking versus Indoor Rowing.

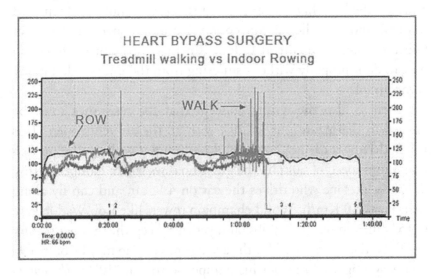

This is the best anti aging tool, as it allows accurate monitored exercise that you can perform at your own level and review, and the motivation comes from the automatic worldwide ranking that Concept2 does for you when you register on the Concept2 personal logbook. Even children get so excited when they register on the Personal logbook of Concept2, and this is a lifelong habit that will stand them in good stead as they eventually age.

The criticism is that the resistance feels so light that it is hard to imagine any benefit from using it. Yet faithful users can still be seen on it at the age of 90, and a 67 year old can rank World #2 against 27 year olds in open age group competition among some 3,000 rowers throughout the World.

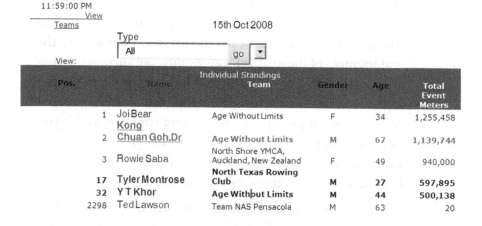

9/15/2008 through
10/15/2008
11:59:00 PM
View
Teams                                    15th Oct 2008
                    Type
                    All                          go
View:

| Pos. | | Name | Team | Gender | Age | Total Event Meters |
|---|---|---|---|---|---|---|
| | 1 | Joi Bear Kong | Age Without Limits | F | 34 | 1,255,458 |
| | 2 | Chuan Goh, Dr | Age Without Limits | M | 67 | 1,139,744 |
| | 3 | Rowie Saba | North Shore YMCA, Auckland, New Zealand | F | 49 | 940,000 |
| | 17 | Tyler Montrose | North Texas Rowing Club | M | 27 | 597,895 |
| | 32 | Y T Khor | Age Without Limits | M | 44 | 500,138 |
| | 2298 | Ted Lawson | Team NAS Pensacola | M | 63 | 20 |

Individual Standings

The thighs of Goeff, the 70 yr old World Champion are the envy of any body builder, but they are seldom shown except by some avid web surfers and lectures on the Benefits of Indoor Rowing who can do a google search for him, under CRASH B winners for >70 around 2004. While many remark that they are not into competition, and only *"Exercise for health"*. It is human to admire the achievements of those who have won in World Open competition, and the standard of health is often measured in the achievements of these few. We imagine these to be the supreme example of health and fitness, and try to emulate them.

The muscles used in Indoor Rowing can be found in the Home page of Concept2 (just do a google search for it), and many other sites, but it will not be reproduced here because of copyright issues.

In my experience from marathon running, looking after countless patients, and training on all the other modes of exercise, this is the recommended mode of exercise for anti aging. The elderly can row in comfort in their own homes, away from:

- The "Free Radicals" and other pollutants that are often blamed for causing the "Aging wrinkles" we see on our skin, and the many types of Cancer that plague modern society. There are already some instruments that claim to measure the level of these pollutants in the atmosphere that have been blamed for causing premature aging and many common diseases. These have not been medically proven, and do not carry the endorsement of the medical community, but their marketing is so strong that many seek them. There is no point in scoring high marks on such a piece of equipment or feeling scared when you score poorly. Just go out and compete, and if you can function well and still beat those half your age, you are in much better shape than that feeble person who may get high scores on this new-fangled instrument.

- The accidents and muggers that we are exposed to when exercising outdoors. We read of so many newspaper reports of those killed or attacked while out for their daily exercise. It makes sense to exercise safely indoors. We do not need the stimulation of the esthetic senses that exercising outdoors offers because modern technology can simulate all this simply with interactive electronic connections. This observation is made by the author who had trained outdoors for years, and run many marathons as well as hiked up some 10,000ft mountains. How many really experience the euphoria of running through a Scotch mist on a secluded mountain ridge? Those who really need this esthetic stimulation can find it in their imagination, and do not need to be exposed to the dangers and discomfort that comes from exercising outdoors.

- The elements such as rain, heat, thirst and lightning that threaten us outside. Only the experience of daily marathon training can teach us this, and we would like those reading this book to learn from our bad memories.

Some love to listen to music while they exercise; some watch the television, and we see so many rowers enjoying their favorite past time while getting their daily quota of exercise. They can even mind the children while exercising.

As we grow older we want to exercise in comfort, and not stress ourselves to suffer from "overstrain" or anything that we cannot control when we exercise away from home. We can find all this when we row indoors on the Indoor Rower. By sitting down, we take the strain off the knees, and instead, strengthen them by the rhythmic motion of every stroke (this duplicates the action of the Continuous Passive Motion machine used after knee replacement). Of course we can combine it with the occasional Golf, Badminton or other games we want to enjoy socially, but if we row daily, we will be fitter and better prepared to enjoy these games without injury.

There is no perfect exercise mode, and there have been many anecdotal reports of misuse of this powerful exercise tool. Training hard with high intensity and constant competition has led to heart arrhythmia in many senior citizens, and we hear of the expensive treatments and suffering they have to undergo. There are also many diseases we are prone to suffer from because we have inherited that tendency from birth, and there seems to be nothing we can do to avoid this. Ultimately, it is the individual who either reaps the benefits or suffers the consequences of his own behavior. We can only suggest an exercise mode, and point out the mistakes that we have learnt either through our own experience or that of others we have followed closely.

The final proof of the pudding is when we look at the small number of healthy senior citizens left exercising above the age of

90. The cover of the Concept2 Personal logbook shows pictures of Ernestine Bayer and John Hodges still competing at Indoor Rowing above the age of 90. The sport they have remained with is Indoor Rowing, and these are at least two examples of the seniors competing internationally at this very physical sport.

## Key Points

- Introduction to the Concept2 Indoor Rower invented by the Dreissigacker brothers
- The rowing stroke prevents Osteoporosis
- Use legs, not arms to generate force, & keep damper setting at "3".
- Muscles used in Indoor Rowing, e.g. 70 year old Goeff
- Healthcare professionals can use Indoor Rower more to rehabilitate patients
- Safety of Indoor Rowing-Walking vs. Indoor Rowing Heart Rate Monitor Tracing
- Advantages of rowing indoors for seniors
- No perfect exercise, but what exercise at 90+?

# 3
# Walking

Let me continue to examine other popular Modes of Exercise.

Brisk walking has been advised by all Doctors as the best mode of exercise, and it is extremely popular and easy to take up. After all we learned to walk after crawling as infants, but is such a vague statement the ultimate advice? What is "brisk" to one may be "slow" to another. I have recorded the heart rate tracings of 2 persons of similar age (above 50).

- One is a weight lifter, and walks at 4+mph on a treadmill for 20+min. with a heart rate averaging >140pm

- The other is a marathon runner who walks the same 4+mph with a heart rate averaging 100bpm.

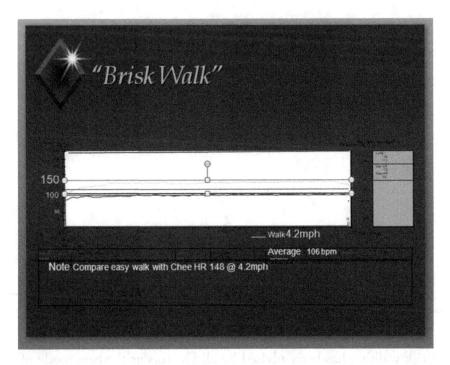

"Brisk Walk"

150
100

____ Walk 4.2mph
Average 106 bpm

Note Compare easy walk with Chee HR 148 @ 4.2mph

 

This illustrates very clearly that what is "brisk" to the sedate is "slow" to the trained and fit, and of little benefit unless practiced for practically the whole day! If you prefer not to use a heart rate monitor, then gauge your exertion level.
"If you can talk without gasping", then the pace is not too fast.

"If you can sing", then you are walking too slowly.

This is the Talk Sing Test [iii].

To be more technical, you can go by the Borg Rating of Perceived Exertion (Borg RPE) test [iv].

This gives descriptive terms for each level of exertion, from 6 or 7 (very very light) to 19 (very very hard) or 20.

Some like to go by the feel of sweating, but in a hot humid environment, you can sweat profusely just sitting down quietly in a chair, and sweating is not a good guide to exercise intensity. If you want to be more objective, invest in a proper heart rate monitor, and you can actually see your heart rate displayed while you exercise. The heart rate range to be in is calculated in many ways, from the simple percentage of the usual calculated maximum heart rate to the complex Karvonen's formula based on the L.Kaminski formula to calculate the maximum heart rate.

Whichever formula is used, do not go rigidly by the calculated value,

The latest Physical Activity Guidelines from the US Physical Activity Guidelines Advisory Committee Report 2009 state:

" The estimated gross energy expenditure needed to achieve weight maintenance following substantial weight loss is about 31Kilocalories per week.... which is equivalent to walking 54 minutes per day at 4 mph pace, **walking 80 minutes per day at 3mph pace**, or jogging 26 min. per day at 6mph.

An oft repeated phrase in the report is **"some is good; more is better"**. This simply means that the more exercise we put in the better it is for our health. The recent guidelines differ from the ACSM Position stand in 1998 in that a specific pace of walking is stated instead of just advising people to exercise for 30 minutes a day. Then we see that the duration of exercise has been more than doubled, seeing that the old recommendation did not have any impact at all on the worsening problem of Obesity these days.

## Walking style

Look at the walkers around you, and observe them closely. There are power walkers, recreational walkers and racewalkers. We have learnt to walk since we progressed to it after crawling as infants, but do we really walk correctly without injury?

The walking style varies from person to person, but is regulated by rules for the racewalker. **USATF Definition**

- Race walking is a progression of steps so taken that the walker makes contact with the ground so that no visible (to the human eye) loss of contact occurs.

- The advancing leg must be straightened (i.e., not bent at the knee) from the moment of first contact with the ground until in the vertical upright position.

The senior recreational walker often complains of knee injuries, whereas the racewalker rarely complains, but just walks on and on, sometimes for 100KM (the Centurions). Isn't it sensible to emulate someone who can walk for 100KM without complaints, rather than someone who walks for around 5KM, complaining all the time that his feet or his knees are killing him?

It gets too technical to train someone to be a racewalker, but basically,

- one foot is always in contact with the ground

- the knee is locked straight from the moment the heel strikes the ground until the rear foot is in the vertical position under the center of the body.

We can see that there is no springing off the ground as in running/jogging, and this prevents the usual injuries associated with runners. The straight knee also gets rid of that knee pain hill climbers, tennis players and those taking up sports always complain of (they proudly wear their knee guards to show that they are "true" sportsmen).

So by taking up the racewalking style of walking, we can move along at a fast pace without suffering from those overuse injuries other exercisers complain about as they age.

There is a technical difference between Race and Power Walking, as the aims are different. In Racewalking the aim is to decrease the resistance, and walk faster. This is achieved by placing the advancing foot 1/3 of the distance in front of the Center of Gravity, while in Power Walking; it is 50% in front. When we plant the advancing foot only 50% in front of the Center of Gravity, we have to work against the resistance it offers to the advancing foot, so by planting it only 30% in front, we encounter less resistance from the foot in front. The Chinese racewalkers have used this technique to put them in the forefront in racewalking, and they can generate a much faster turnover to walk at above 200 strides per minute.

We see so many exercisers walking while holding on to dumb bells (purportedly to increase the resistance and "burn more Calories"). This cramps the walking style, and contributes to walking injuries, so that we often see these same Power Walkers bandaged up while they continue their daily exercise without these same dumb bells, or constantly complaining of shoulder aches and pains. They have chosen to learn this the hard way, from their personal experience, and we can only point this out to those who want to hear. Just walk faster or longer if you need to burn more Calories, and don't hold on to dumb bells.

There are also those who teach powerful pumping of the arms. But if you watch a racewalker, you will see how effortlessly he walks. It is only when you learn all those drills he undergoes that you understand how complicated it can get. It is important to walk naturally, and not get bogged down with too much pedantic instruction.

This reference to champions is also applicable to the average exerciser, and though many protest "we walk only for health", we can learn to walk more efficiently from these great champions. There may be a lot of reference to "recreational walking", "walking for leisure", and many other titles, as if these are distinct styles of walking. The important thing is to look at the end result, and see who can walk more efficiently and enjoy this mode of exercise way into old age.

## The Great Outdoors

Many people like to walk in the parks because they enjoy the beauty of natural surroundings. But nowadays it is frightening to hear of those attacked while out for their morning exercise. Is it worth this risk while trying to get our daily exercise? There is a safer alternative- to exercise indoors, yet this is spurned by many. Mall walking is a growing form of exercise in the Houston malls that have been marked out for distance, and seniors can be seen doing their daily exercise in the safety and comfort of the air conditioned malls.

Walking also leads to hiking, and many macho exercisers seek out the steepest hills to climb because they feel that walking on level ground "does not make them sweat". They tell us of the sense of accomplishment when they summit a difficult climb up a mountain, and show pictures of the glorious view from up there. I always ask them if they have been competitive enough to win at any walking races, and invariably they cannot show any medals or cite any wins to support their so-called competitiveness. Racewalking on level ground certainly makes you sweat, and the correct technique leads to less strain on the body than walking on undulating ground. I take part in endurance races lasting 12 to 24 hours, and always measure the energy expended during such races. I don't think this subjective sensation of elation during such climbs does as much to contribute towards anti aging as the consistent walking we do daily.

From this accurate data obtained, we can easily compare the energy output from such endurance races and exercising indoors in the gym. There is no use guessing at this, and the conclusion is that walking does not burn as much energy as racewalking or Indoor Rowing. This comparison should convince anyone of the benefits of walking if properly done, and how it compares to the other two modes of exercise mentioned- racewalking and Indoor Rowing.

The American Record for racewalking 1 mile is 5:40 seconds, while a Connecticut lady racewalker has walked 1 mile in just over 6 minutes. This compares with the famous World Running record, where Roger Bannister managed to run 1 mile in 4 min.

But the average person walks at the pace of 16 min. for 1 mile, and to even cover 1 mile in 11:30 seconds, it needs much training and good technique. As a rough guide, it takes about 11 minutes for the average person to walk 1 round of the lower loop (0.92KM) of the Penang Botanical Gardens, a common exercise spot for those who like to experience natural surroundings in this tropical isle. A good speed is 16 minutes to cover the 0.8 miles from gate to gate along the ridge of the Canyon Lake dam in Texas.

The latest example is an improvement of 19.2% in three days.

The time taken to racewalk along the summit of Canyon Lake was compared on 3 successive days. The distance from gate to gate is written down as 0.8 miles.

- 6/27/06….. 52 minutes or 12:45 seconds to cover 0.8 miles
- 6/29/06….50:52 seconds. This gives a racewalking pace of 15.88 min. per mile. It may appear fast among the slow recreational walkers around, but measured in absolute minutes per mile, it is certainly slow, and really drives home the message that pace must be measured in absolute terms.

This was done at the age of 67, and when it is repeated next year, it will show if anti aging really works with exercise. That will really track the effects of aging.

These examples are to show that we should never guess our distances or walking pace, and it is no trouble at all to measure it accurately on a 400 meter school running track or other measured circuit. Even the malls are marked out for distance in Houston, and a class of exercisers has sprouted, known as the "Mall Walkers" who form their own Clubs – "The Mall Walker's Club", recognizing those who have managed to reach milestones in their daily walking. It certainly does a lot to the ego to be recognized for your achievements, and I believe this helps a lot towards providing motivation towards exercising and maintaining the consistency of exercise.

## Walking aids:

<u>The Treadmill</u>- this adorns every gym, and ideally can help those who want to continue walking indoors without being exposed to the sun or muggers. I used to train for marathons by running for 5 to 6 hours on the treadmill, breaking every half an hour run with a drink or a banana. But we must never touch or hold on to the treadmill rails if we want to keep track of the calories burnt- they have been calibrated without the user holding on to the rails. Some users have suffered from shoulder injuries from hanging on too long to the treadmill rails (One had to undergo an operation), and the estimation used is 120 Calories per mile covered on the flat. The treadmill is also not built to withstand long hours of usage at the maximum grade of incline these hangers-on walk/run at. As a result, many of the treadmills at gyms and clubs often break down.

Many treadmills have heart rate sensors built into a handle you briefly touch, but these are always covered with a film of sweat, and are inaccurate when compared to the heart rate displayed when a heart rate monitor belt is properly worn on the chest. It is a gimmick put in by those who design equipment, and I do not recommend them over the properly worn heart rate transmitter belt.

Watch out for foot pain because the treadmill belt moves towards your feet, and can cause pain when the foot lands on it. Other than that, the treadmill is a good piece of equipment to use if these simple rules are followed.

For athletes they can train on the treadmill by alternating intervals of fast running (about 40 seconds at 10mph) followed by long runs of 3 hours at 6 or 7mph. The unfit heart bypass (CABG) patient can even benefit from walking slowly at 2kmph without holding on to the treadmill rails. The other trick is to locate the treadmill facing a mirror so that you look straight ahead into the reflection of your feet far away, and will never fall down. Never look to the side when walking/running on a treadmill, because you will fall down (I have fallen down a few times when distracted and looking to the side). The most important thing is never to hold on to the treadmill rails and fool you into seeing the calories moving so fast.

Walking Poles- are a new walking accessory that helps a walker to enjoy walking farther. They have to be properly held and swung rhythmically when walking, and actually burn more calories than when walking without them. But you have to wear a heart rate monitor to keep track of the calories burnt this way.

They have been further developed into the climbing poles and ski poles that are specialty accessories. The former help in climbing, especially downhill, and the latter are part of ski equipment.

Further information can be found by a simple "google" search on the web.

## Pedometers

This is the subject of a lecture itself, but if the reader is interested, we can talk a bit about them. They are simple devices attached to the belt that accurately record every step you walk throughout the day. Many such devices have been evaluated, and in some the accuracy may vary from 4,000 to 14,000 steps for the same activity in the day. So it is important to use the pedometer that is truly accurate, and the Yamax has come out tops in the scientific studies conducted. The recommendation (by the Japanese) is 10,000 steps in 1 day

If the average step is 2.6 ft, this works out to 26,500 ft.

Since 1 mile =5,280ft, a simple calculation will show that this comes to about 5 miles a day,

The average energy consumption is 120 Calories a mile. So this works out to about 600 Calories burnt a day if you walk 5 miles according to the recommendation of 10,000 steps a day. If you walk slowly these 10,000 steps a day, you will burn 600 Calories a day, or 4,200 Calories a week. Compare this to the figure of 2,000 Calories a week given by Paffenbarger in his Yale Alumni study, and we are right on track.

Does walking really help in anti aging? While we see many struggling to follow their "Doctor's orders" to "Walk for Health", we have to look at the practical issues. The very people it is supposed to help- the elderly are often struggling with knee problems, and have great difficulty walking. So what is the point of recommending this mode of exercise that causes them so much pain and difficulty? This is a very common ailment, and it affects the sedentary who think they have been practicing a healthy lifestyle by using the stairs instead of the elevator.

Theoretically this may sound good advice, but try telling that to the average sedate 80 year old, and (s)he will loudly protest that it is impossible to walk. My "cover" girl could easily walk the 2 miles from the UN building to the New York Metropolitan Art Museum when she was 78, but now at 88, she cannot walk even half that distance without a knee guard to diminish the pain, but she can row on the Indoor Rower for 40 minutes without discomfort! There are other modes of exercise more suited to the elderly, and we have to be practical about it.

# Key Points

- Brisk walking is relative to fitness level
- Talk/Gasp/Sing test. Borg RPE scale
- DHHS activity guidelines
- Recreational vs. racewalking
- Walking outdoors and hiking; use of walking aids and poles
- Treadmill walking
- Pedometers for monitoring
- Is walking really suitable for anti aging?

# 4
# Swimming

This has been proclaimed the ideal exercise by those who swim, (and I took it up at the age of 5, while my father swam daily for >65 years). It certainly benefits the cardiovascular system, and develops the shoulders and legs used for propelling you through the water.

While swimming you float on the water (reducing your weight in air of some 70Kg to the weight of some 2Kg in water- I discovered this fact when testing my own Total Body Fat by Total Water Immersion at the University of Lacrosse, Wisconsin). While this takes the weight off your knees, feet and hips, it makes you practically weightless (like an Astronaut), and we know how these great athletes suffer from Osteoporosis when they stay too long in Space. I had the good fortune to meet up with Peter Snell (the great NZ athlete who once held 8 World records at middle distance running around the Tokyo and Rome Olympics). He now works as Associate Professor in Cardiology in Dallas, Texas, and researches on Osteoporosis in NASA astronauts. He finds that treadmills, stationary bikes and weights cannot help these Astronauts, while Indoor Rowing prevents Osteoporosis when they stay long in Space [v]. He has the latest "Bone Elasticity Machine" that measures improvement in the bone long before the much touted "Bone turnover markers" or "DEXA machine".

The weightlessness experienced in Space is total, and demonstrates in a much shorter time what we experience when swimming. We do not need a lifetime of swimming to show up the Osteoporosis that a stint in Space demonstrates in these fantastic athletes. There will be those who argue that swimming is nothing compared to Space travel, but is it worth wasting a whole lifetime on a mode of exercise when you can see the accelerated result right in front of you. Better still, you do not have to suffer from the Osteoporosis-just read about it, and decide if that is what you want or can avoid.

Swimming helps those with Asthma too because of the humid air they breathe in, and the regulated rhythmic strokes swimming demands. Many World swimming champs suffer from Asthma. It builds up the cardiovascular system with slow progressive training, and develops patience because you cannot interact socially with anyone when your head is immersed in the water. It also takes the load off the knees, and is good for those suffering from Osteoarthritis. While the force of marketing has made most people think of Glucosamine/Chondroitin, Osteoporosis should be associated with non-weight bearing exercise that allows us to move our knees and develop the muscles around them. This is truly economical, and takes us off this dependence on medicine to treat our ailments that may be due to disuse and degeneration.

Many rehabilitation experts advise swimming to rehabilitate from musculoskeletal injuries (and many references to this can be easily found on the web). But to swimmers like us, it is not practical. I have experienced the excruciating pain shooting up the spine when trying to stay afloat. So many muscles are called into play, and unless you move those muscles at a high intensity you will find yourself sinking into the water.

Swimming develops a certain skill and dedication that builds up character in a person, and will contribute much to his later life.

One final point about swimming is that all swimmers have a higher total body fat content than others. This is because the body is always immersed in a low temperature, and the natural reaction is to accumulate more subcutaneous fat to insulate it from the cold. It is only the competitive swimmers in training who burn thousands of Calories a day who manage to stay slim, because their output far exceeds their input, and the Calorie balance stays negative, like Michael Phelps [vi].

I recommend swimming for the discipline it develops, and the strong cardiovascular training effect, as well as the skill learnt. However, it is not the complete exercise, and swimmers must learn to lift weights or find something else to do to round up their exercise and prevent this tendency towards Osteoporosis that prolonged weightlessness can lead to. I have been associated with swimming for more than half a century, and find that old swimmers all become crippled when they approach 80 because of the Osteoporosis they develop. The silent multiple fractures and healing of the spine they suffer from causes narrowing of the spinal canal, and squeezes the spinal cord, thus preventing the signals from the brain from reaching the legs, and crippling them. This is a common ailment not realized by swimmers until they suffer from it late in their lives, and it is too late to reverse the process.

Most swimmers develop the mentality that they have found the perfect exercise, and have no time for anything else; so they swim on until they become crippled for the last years of their lives. There is no Quality of Life left, and it is such a pity when there are other forms of exercise they could have taken up together with their swimming that could have led them to a better life.

## Key Points

- Personal experience with swimming
- Swimming and Osteoporosis in Old Age
- Swimming helps with Asthma
- Swimming exacerbates pain in rehabilitation
- Higher Total Body Fat in Swimming
- Swimming alone is not the ideal exercise for seniors.

# 5

# Running

This is an excellent form of exercise for controlling the body weight and developing the cardiovascular system. Many books have been written on it, and the "Bible" of running can be found in Tim Noakes' *Lore of Running,* a 400+ page book that has run into its 4<sup>th</sup> edition.[vii]

The child runs freely (and happily) in his playground after mastering the skill of walking, but the avid exerciser jogs slowly along, with that long-suffering look on his face. We must learn to be child-like, and enjoy whatever we are doing. The dynamics of running are so simple, but when we break it down scientifically it becomes complicated, with the gait analysis, *the foot-strike, and the spring off the foot as well as the jarring forces on the knee and the pronation and supination* that all contribute to the many injuries the runner always complains of. Why must something so simple and natural become so complicated and expensive?

Yes, it can become very expensive when you have to see the Doctor or Podiatrist repeatedly for that troublesome leg injury, or when you have to pay increasingly more for that treadmill that used to cost only $1,500, but can now cost up to $30,000 (for the HP Cosmo). When you calibrate a $2,000 treadmill you find that the speed can vary by 10% from the true calculated speed for that length of treadmill belt. Then again, when you see those gym rats holding on to the treadmill, and galloping along with the maximum grade, while *hanging on for dear life to the rails*, you cease to wonder why they stay so fat in spite of the thousands of Calories flashing on the display. When will they ever learn that those Calorie readouts cease to have any more meaning the moment they *hold on to the rails*? These machines have been calibrated with people running freely on them. The moment your hands touch the rails, this becomes assisted, and the display ceases to have any more meaning. I have tested a subject on it, using the Bruce Protocol, the commonest stress test done. When he did not hold on to the treadmill rails, he could last only 12 minutes, putting him at stage 4 (an average fit person),  but when he held on to the rails, he lasted 18 minutes, putting him at stage VI (a superior athlete). The assistance was unbelievable, and would have resulted in the wrong classification if we had allowed him to hold on to the treadmill rails.

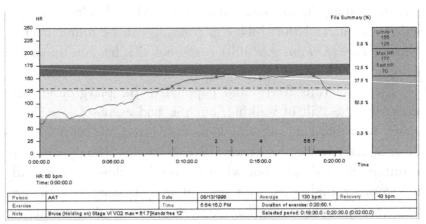

## Outdoor Running

The runner in training for marathons enjoys the outdoors, and runs from the darkness of 5am through the dawn, until it gets a bit too hot and humid to continue. Where else can you hear the loud call of the *Koel* bird, or see the beauty of the rising run, and feel the coolness of dawn as you run with the wind? That is one of the joys the endurance runner experiences, and not the showing off that he has run a full hour on the treadmill, or 50 rounds of the field under the hot sun. It is one of the motivational tools that keep him going on in a discipline many would consider boring. Many people talk of the esthetic stimulation they get from exercising outdoors, but do they really listen to nature? Take it from one who has run 10 marathons, and trained every morning and evening for these events. Have you really listened to the serenade of the early morning birds as they sing out from their nests to prepare for the beautiful day ahead, or listened to the noisy chatter of these same birds at dusk as they return to roost? Have you run through a light drizzle and fog along a secluded mountain ridge? Once again we hear exercisers claiming to be runners, and despising racewalkers or those taking up other modes of exercise. If they have truly experienced these moments, then they can claim to be among those who really appreciate the beauty of nature. The experience is out of this world, but there is a time to enjoy all these, and we must focus on anti aging and find the best mode of exercise that suits us, and will achieve long lasting results.

## Running downhill

*Running downhill causes knee injuries.* This is another myth the exercisers believe, and they try to avoid doing so because of the "knee injury" this is supposed to cause. But competitive runners often train running downhill, (to improve the cadence), and many of us recreational runners have run down Penang Hill (a favorite site for hikers on this tropical island hill- about 5KM long and 700m high) for about half an hour without suffering any knee injury for decades. It is true that the pressure on the articulating surfaces in the knee is increased in normal downhill running. But we see martial arts experts running lightly over silk cloth (as in the Beijing Olympics Opening ceremony) or even *taufu*, and we skip so lightly downhill that there is never any discomfort felt in the knee joints. Many have been converted to downhill running, and returned to their favorite sport of hill climbing after rehabilitating from the knee injuries they had sustained through their old style of running. If properly done, downhill running is so enjoyable, and we should not listen to those who look horrified at us flying downhill with ease.

Running is enjoyable, but the motivation to keep on running is fuelled by company and competition. You train harder and look forward to running when you do so with good company, and runners often group together with colorful names like "The Mad Bunch", or the "Old and Young". I used to enter every fun run, and the mild competition from the pack stimulates you to improve, as you find yourself overtaking familiar faces in successive runs. But we can never emulate the Kenyans, and there is not much fun finding yourself at the back of the pack, or not winning any medals. However, the benefits of running far outweigh this trivial point, and you gain good health, as you find your medical and drug bills going down, and your weight control is so easy, as you eat all you like. You enjoy "Runner's trots" (where you find you can move your bowels regularly at will) and never have to worry about constipation. Sleep is never a problem, and you wonder why some people become so dependent on sleeping pills.

The average running speed is a 10 minute mile, or the marathon (26 miles) in 4h 20min.

This compares with the World record marathon 2h 03:59 min. run at a pace of 4.8473 min., or 4:43.7 min. per mile consistently for >26 miles.

Most of us are comfortable jogging along at a 12 min./mile pace (marathon in 5 hr 11 min.).

One complete round of the lower loop of the Botanical Gardens in Penang has been measured with the surveyor's wheel to be 920 m, and the loop around the Water Lily Pond measures 232 m, while the upper loop (where the car can drive around) measures 1.6 KM, and the loop up to the reservoir measures 1.9 Km. If you can run the lower loop (0.92 KM) of the Gardens in 4:20 seconds repeatedly, that is very good time. Some marathon runners have done 45 rounds in their training sessions. Again, these are favorite training grounds in this tropical isle, and examples of how you can accurately measure your running pace wherever you may be.

*Interval Running* is a good way of training for races, as it gives you SPEED ENDURANCE, and does not strain the heart and musculo-skeletal system as much as running lsd. Too much long slow distance (lsd) running deadens the muscles, and prevents the springing off the ground you see in energetic young runners. It grooves in a slow pace. So the elderly runner must run intervals to avoid this staleness that creeps in from too much slow running for long distances.

Besides this, *Endorphin release* usually happens when you run fast intervals, with some rest interval in between. This is the "Zone" we all seek, when you get the feeling of exhilaration from sudden bursts of speed while running. These *opioids* are naturally stimulated to be released from the brain, and make you feel good and want to continue running. So try to incorporate "Interval training" into your running schedule, and it will not only promote "anti aging", but keep you running and enjoying every minute of it.

Run, but pay attention to other muscles (of the upper body) that may atrophy, and to your bones that may suffer from Osteoporosis (many a runner has suffered from the broken bones of Osteoporosis). Women, especially may suffer from the Female Athlete Triad (that is not limited to the young athlete), and must beware of that obsessive compulsion that leads to Anorexia Nervosa, Osteoporosis and all those problems that may arise from behavior and excessive dieting. This condition is caused by suppression of Estrogen secretion by these women so that they suffer from Osteoporosis that leads to stress fractures.

## Key Points

- Run freely, and enjoy it like a child
- Don't hold on to rails when running on the treadmill
- Esthetic beauty of nature experienced when running
- Run in good company and mild competition
- Running downhill is bad for the knees- myth
- Measure exact speed when training and exercising for general health
- Avoid Dietary problems like Anorexia Nervosa
- Complement running with muscle development to prevent injuries

# 6
# Weight Training

This is the delight of personal trainers, and many see the gym as the place for only building up muscles. While this is true to a certain extent, we must remember that it is the total exercise that is of benefit in anti aging. In the gym there are many different types of weight equipment. It is generally advisable to use free weights rather than machine weights. Free weights call into play other accessory muscles to stabilize the body, and this is more natural than the isolated muscles the machines focus on. Body builders always stress anatomical muscle definition so that the individual muscles stand out, but for anti aging purposes this is totally unnecessary, and looks ugly to the elderly. Besides it gets so expensive to develop one of these specialized machines when a set of dumb bells or barbells can be used for so many sets of exercises and prevent muscle imbalance. Muscle imbalance must be corrected with the exercises for opposing muscles.

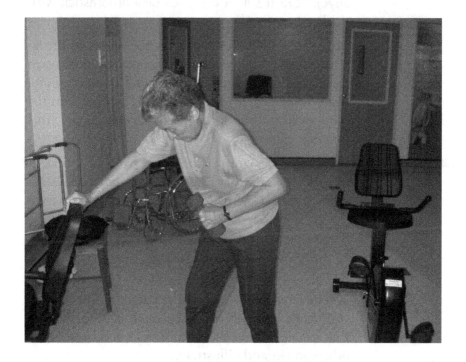

1. **"Triceps Kickback"**, done with 2Kg weights here is the perfect exercise to develop the back of the upper arm that is usually flabby in the elderly. It corrects the imbalance from the biceps that are located in the front of the upper arm, and that are more often used from carrying things such as groceries. In the gym a lot of stress is placed on development of the biceps.

2. **"Wand Exercise"**, illustrated so elegantly by our 80+ year old model who has been suffering from Osteoarthritis for more than 20 years. We hear of many seniors having knee pain who cannot climb steps to the mahjong room to enjoy their favorite pastime. Many seniors scoff at the "Wand exercises" because they think it is too simple for them, but the many advantages stated below will convince them to try it.

- Firstly, the weight of the "wand" is very light, and anyone can lift it. It can even be a broomstick with the head removed.

- Next, balance is developed, as the alternate lifting of the arms and legs develops co-ordination between them, and forces the senior to stand on one leg at a time. Some people even play music, and perform the motions in time with the music; for most people this makes it enjoyable.

- If the exercises are performed in front of a sofa, it is perfectly safe, because (s)he can fall backwards safely into the sofa if (s)he loses balance. We have a powerful exercise tool here for the aging and those recovering from strokes.

- In my experience "Wand Exercises" need to be introduced to really help the elderly instead of the "Chair Exercises" we see being taught all the time in churches and other senior centers. It is time to adopt this mode of exercise that my 80+ year old and many others so elegantly illustrate.

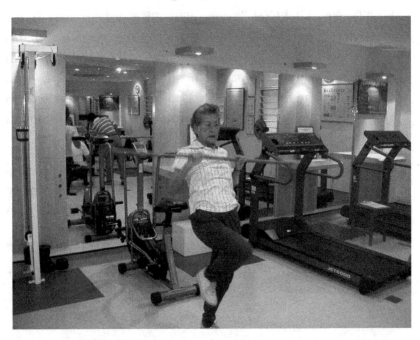

3. **Squats** The elderly find that the thigh muscles are the first to weaken, and we often find those in their sixties have difficulty getting up from a squatting position. Some cannot even climb a high step such as getting into a van. The simplest squat is against your own body weight, and many practice this with their backs against the wall, repeating it as many times as they can. Good marketing and pride in ancient exercise has made this one of the traditional exercises, and we are often called copycats when we do this simple exercise. The next step is to do a one-legged squat, tucking one leg behind the knee, and repeating as many squats as you can, then going down as low as you can. If you can dance like a Cossack, then you are really in good shape, but we need not try to emulate them if we are only into anti aging exercises. Trying to do the impossible sometimes discourages some people from trying at all, and they complain that exercise is so hard.

4. Step ups. For the feeble and elderly with weak knees they can do step-ups on a low step. The sequence is very important, so that alternate legs are raised every time, and this has to be practiced repeatedly until it becomes automatic, and grooved into the mind. Then, they can progress on to a higher step, until the thigh is horizontal to the ground, and the lower leg makes an angle of 90 degrees with it (about a foot high step) The final step (for the stronger ones) is to wear a knapsack, and put in a few books  to load the legs and try the step-ups.

5. Padded tin and Straight Leg lifts. For the very weak, and those suffering from weak knees, they can put a padded round tin behind the knees, and push each of them down (as well as digging in the heels) while lying flat. This is best shown by a practical demonstration. After this, they can progress on to straight leg lifts, wearing an ankle weight of 1lb, then 2 lbs, and even 5 lbs, while lifting the straight leg off a bed or couch. This takes considerable patience, and

the feeble must not try to lift heavier weights too soon, then complain of knee pain, and that the exercise is useless.

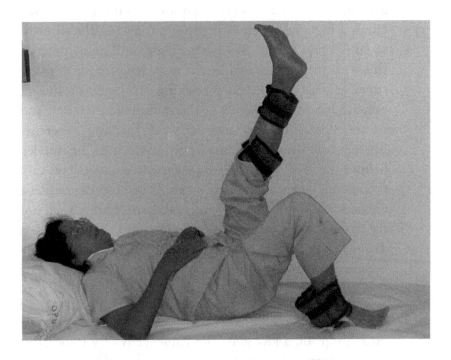

## Important observations about Weight Training

1. People do not have the **patience** to perform the many repetitions and sets needed to get results. Sprinters like the late Flo Jo have very well developed muscles through weight training, but the average exerciser does not need serious weight training. Just accept the "wand exercises" and simple dumb bells and barbells for anti aging purposes.

2. There are some senior athletes who think that these exercises described above are too **elementary** for them. "Squat jumps, jumping jacks, burpees and shuttle runs" are some exercises they may consider. However, these are very demanding exercises recommended only for the athlete in training, and not for the average exerciser.

3. Weight training prevents **Osteoporosis**. But it must be properly guided. This was the theory put forward by Rubin and Lanyon when they said that there is a certain Minimum Effective Strain (MES) that has to be exceeded to stimulate the Osteoblasts to grow new bone. This means that the bone is deformed by a certain percentage, exactly measured by a strain gauge. They performed elegant experiments on animals that cannot be duplicated on man, and this was even quoted in the American College of Sports Medicine Position Stand on Osteoporosis in the late 1990s. The closest this has been substantiated is the work by Kevin Vincent and R. Braith in their *"Resistance exercise and bone turnover by elderly men and women (*MSSE Vol. 42 No.1 Jan 2002 Pg. 17-23). I have also worked with many seniors who have reversed their Osteoporosis without any medication, but purely through exercise. Good examples are our cover girls, our 88 year old and our 66 year old who have both been closely monitored with DEXA bone studies. The best example is our 76 year old with the fractured ankle who recovered completely to win medals.

4. **BP rise in Weight Training.** We are very careful about Blood Pressure control, and nowadays Doctors talk about lowering goals (BP levels) in their quest for better health and prevention of Disease. But it has been found that during exercise the BP can rise, and in 1 research study, it has been found that the simple leg press that is so common in most gyms can even raise the BP to 480/350.[viii] This will horrify most exercisers especially when we hear of so many who have died so suddenly of burst cerebral aneurysms or other weak blood vessels they have been born with. That is why it is so important to lift weights the correct way, and to exhale while exerting to try to reduce this BP rise. If we were aware of this danger, we seniors would be careful about heavy weight training, and leave it to the hardcore body builders

and professional sportsmen who balance this risk against the big bucks they earn.

## Key Points

- Free weights better than machines in gym
- Triceps kickback to correct muscle imbalance
- Wand exercises, squats, step-ups, straight leg lifts to strengthen knees
- Jumping jacks, burpees are aerobic exercises for the senior athlete
- Weight training prevents Osteoporosis
- Blood Pressure rise in weight training

# 7

# Cycling

Cycling, whether outdoors or on the stationary bike in the gym does give results, and the person with the highest measured VO2max in the World is the cyclist, Miguel Indurain (at 95ml O2 per Kg per min.)[ix].

So the legends spread as a way of explaining why one person wins consistently. It happened with Miguel Indurain, a Spaniard who won five consecutive tours in the 1990's. Mr. Indurain's VO2 max, according to a widespread rumor, was 95 milliliters per kilogram of body weight per minute, a level so high it is unheard of. The real number was 78, Dr. Coyle said, but researchers who tested Mr. Indurain were reluctant to put the true figure in their paper for fear of demolishing the Indurain myth.

The criticism has been made that this is too unrealistic a level for the average exerciser or senior to reach, but the fact remains that people are only dazzled by the achievements of the greatest champions, often dominating dinner conversations with the latest achievements of these great champions they have read about in the news media. This has been stated before in Chapter 2 on Indoor Rowing just after the chart of the Fall Rowing challenge results, and we can see so many people watching these World champions in action on the television Sports Channel.

The average cyclist is often fitter than those who exercise on other machines. He looks young, slim and fit. Cross country skiers may come fairly close, but even great runners like the legendary Peter Snell only had a $VO_{2\ max}$ of 70 at their peak. This information is easily available on the web

To the average exerciser cycling is a quick way to get fit, enjoy the outdoors, and socialize. The leg muscles and heart get most of the training effects, and this benefits most people who exercise "*just for health*". One does not have to compete or even to emulate the great champion cyclists to benefit from it.

For the seniors, I would recommend the stationary recumbent bike instead of the upright stationary bike. These are some of the reasons why cycling indoors on the recumbent bike is better than outdoors:

1. It is much safer to cycle indoors on the stationary bike, as many cyclists and triathletes have been known to be knocked down by cars while training outdoors.

2. In the gym, the recumbent bike has a padded seat instead of a saddle. This is much more comfortable, and gets rid of that troublesome numbness in the crotch that plagues most long distance cyclists (and sometimes makes them impotent, so say many triathletes).

3. Lying back on a recumbent seat with back support also gets rid of that troublesome backache that affects most cyclists when they have to crouch to hold the handle. We often see exercisers choosing the upright over the recumbent bike because they think they will be labeled soft (called a wimp) if they use the recumbent bike.

It has been my observation that many regular exercisers do not get the desired benefits they seek from cycling, and I will now discuss why this is so.

- <u>Proper cycling Technique</u>

  o There is a minimum pedal rate of around 74rpm that must be maintained while cycling [x]. This does not only apply to competitive cyclists, but also to the average exercise or the person undergoing rehabilitation for injuries.

We see many stationary cyclists in the gym who are pedaling along slowly around 20rpm while reading a book. Is the book more interesting or the cycling? They should focus on one thing, and that is the cycling they are doing.

  o Cyclists are also very particular about the saddle height, and meticulously measure it. This has to do with the straightening of the knee and proper application of power when pedaling. In fact the pro bicycle shop is where you can get the most technical advice from the qualified and experienced cyclists there.

  o Another point is that cyclists have to push down hard with each leg (often using the up going pedal to pull upwards and lessen the load on the foot that is driving the wheels forward). Most cyclists are unaware of this added assistance from the up going foot.

  o Pushing down hard with each leg often worsens knee pain, and that is why we see so many cyclists suffering from knee pain who don't get any better after years of cycling that has been ordered by the healthcare practitioner.

<u>Heart Rate Monitoring and automatic power output</u>

  o Most stationary bikes have a heart rate monitor incorporated into them. The sensor must be properly positioned and screened to prevent false high readings from appearing on the display, otherwise the heart rate fluctuates wildly, and does not guide us whether to pedal harder or to slow down.

  o However, there is a feature where you set the heart rate you want (in a properly screened machine), and the resistance of the pedal automatically adjusts itself up or down to maintain this heart rate that you have set. This is important for those with heart conditions who do not want to exert themselves too hard. This feature is possible with the electromagnetic clutch found in high end machines like the Lode Excalibur, Lode Corival or the Trotter or Cybex; but cheap mechanical friction stationary bikes are often used in spinning classes, and these depend very much on the cadence (rpm) used for cycling. .

o We also have the road racing bike mounted on a stationary rack that is like the treadmill to the runner. This is used by senior triathletes who still want to complete, and is certainly safer than training outdoors for them. You can cycle at full speed, but still not go anywhere. This allows you to train indoors through all the gears, and at any speed you like, safe from the, pollution, the mad traffic or the elements outside.

## Special Bikes

Mountain bikes are special bikes built for the sport of mountain biking, and there are many groups of such cyclists who enjoy cycling and exploring hill tracks. These are sturdy bikes with multiple gears, and some enjoy cycling up the steep Penang Hill (on the lowest and most mechanically efficient gear) while others enjoy exploring the tracks of many hills in the most ecologically friendly manner.

BMX bikes are used by cyclists training for Extreme games, and we see these cyclists dressed in their protective gear (for the knees and elbows) maneuvering the tough circuits with all their trick cycling.

Some cyclists even wear special shoes such as "clip-ons" that clip on magnetically or into a slot to the base of the pedal. This gives a good fit to assist in the up going pull, and new cyclists have been seen to fall down when they cannot pull out their feet fast enough when they come to a stop.

All the bikes used outdoors need the protective helmet that has been designated compulsory for cyclists in some countries. There are also the padded shorts all cyclists use especially for long rides like the 170mile Trans Florida cycle race.

There is even the kidney-shaped seat to cushion your buttocks, and the camel (a water-containing bladder on your back, with a long straw to your lips) to feed you with water without any interruption to your cycling

Spinning Classes are found in many gyms that use special stationary upright bikes. Exercisers enjoy regular spinning classes where they are led along imaginary courses by the personal trainer who works them through a good sweat.

## Relevance of Cycling to anti aging

1. I have also come across many elderly cyclists who complain that after a hip replacement, they just cannot lift one leg high enough to pedal. When they finally manage to do so, the weak leg just cannot pedal at all.

2. We also see so many seniors with knee replacements who try to rehabilitate on the bicycle, because they have been put on it by rehab staff who believe that cycling is the only low impact exercise suitable for rehabilitating the knees. However, I have observed that they do not show much improvement after many months of cycling, and still complain of weak and stiff knees. This ages them considerably, and they are unable to enjoy the quality life they were used to before.

3. I would like to recommend cycling for the cardiovascular fitness it develops for the seniors, but they should always use the recumbent bike, because it supports the back, and also for the reasons I have stated in the comparison between recumbent and upright bikes.

4. The cycle also does not give any exercise to the upper body. Instead, it often gives rise to backache and weak shoulders and arms. So if you must cycle, do some weight training or some other mode to round up your exercise.

5. The ultimate piece of advice is that cycling outdoors is dangerous, and many a senior athlete has been killed by a road accident, thus giving him no chance to age at all, no matter how fit or healthy he has been keeping himself. Some have only been maimed, and this certainly ages them fast, robbing them of the quality life they have been seeking, and cutting down their life span.

## Key Points

- Cycling outdoors versus cycling indoors
- Advantages of the recumbent bike over the upright bike
- Proper cycling technique
- Heart Rate monitoring
- Special bikes
- Relevance of cycling to anti aging

# 8
# The Cross Trainer

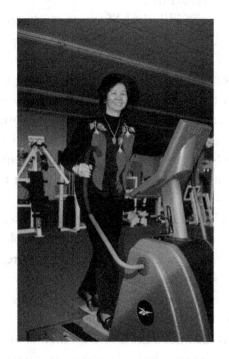

The Cross Trainer, more accurately known as the Elliptical Machine, is one of the more popular pieces of gym aerobic equipment, and has spawned a money-making cash cow in the equipment industry. It is supposed to be the ultimate non-weight bearing exercise that burns large amounts of energy, and not surprisingly, rehabilitation professionals favor it. It seems so easy to get on to an Elliptical machine for a short spell and furiously move your arms and legs, then watch those Calories flashing by on the display. However, after a few weeks on this, you begin to suffer aches and pains from places you never knew existed, and your body shape and weight stay more or less the same. Gym users request for this machine because the marketing is extremely good, and this probably helps to popularize the machine. It is just like line dancing and the traditional Eastern exercises that have a very large following, but one must look at the results. When we look at it objectively, people like to use this machine because they want to keep up with the Jones's. It is fashionable to be on the cross trainer, and you won't look out of place in the gym if you exercise on this machine.

When you use the Elliptical Machine, you need to perform an artificial motion that does not train you for any specific sport, and the movement of the arms and legs is so large and unnatural that it puts a strain on the back and shoulder, leading to backache and shoulder pain. I have observed this in the many patients I watched struggling to exercise on it in many gyms. The mechanical parts also wear out quite fast, and private users (as well as gym owners) have to pay a lot for its wear and tear and maintenance. The Calorie readout is also questionable, and it may be difficult to calibrate such a machine.

So the Cross Trainer may be fashionable to use, but ultimately, does it give the results it promises, and are people still exercising on it when they reach the elderly age of 70 or more? The brave boy frankly revealed the real truth that *"The Emperor wore no clothes"* when everyone else was convinced otherwise; this is the analogy I would like to draw to the Cross Trainer.

I would not recommend the Cross Trainer for anti aging because it is hard on the knees and the back, and users often suffer from these injuries, while they do not lose weight or look any younger or healthier after exercising on it. I just met a friend who was wondering why he is not getting any results in spite of exercising so often on the cross trainer and supposedly burning so many Calories. Instead of sparing the knees and strengthening the back, especially for the seniors, the cross trainer may be aggravating the pain in these parts.

## Key Points

- Cross trainer very popular & fashionable because of good marketing.
- People like to take up popular exercises without caring about the long-term results.
- Many injuries from using the cross trainer

# 9
# Rehabilitation

This is a chapter that needs to be included because it shows how many ordinary people  have become champions after rehabilitating from some injury.

## 1. Florence- High Blood Pressure + Cervical Spondylosis

These are common conditions that would have prematurely aged a person, and one would never have believed this true story, but there are medals and certificates to show it.

Florence had high BP, above 160/100, and was put on the powerful drug-Fortzaar by a doctor for two years. She faithfully followed the doctor's advice several years ago, and there was some improvement. Then she took up Indoor Rowing regularly five to seven times a week, and recorded her BP many times without taking the medication. Lo and behold, she has not been on any medication now for the past 2 years, and her BP has consistently been below 120/80 (monitored and recorded regularly).

This is a true story, and totally against the current medical advice that once you have high BP, you must be on medication for life. You get thoroughly convinced that the effects of high BP will only show up after several years, and in the mean time you have to suffer the side effects of the medication. Perhaps this advice may change in the next generation, when it becomes unfashionable to tolerate the adverse side effects of medication when Lifestyle Modification can be just as effective to control BP.

The Cervical Spondylosis diagnosed by a Radiologist, all disappeared when she did isometric neck exercises and took up Indoor Rowing. Instead of being sidelined, she became the champion at indoor Rowing for 4 successive years, beating people 10 years younger. We have pictures of her during her younger days to demonstrate the effects of Exercise on anti aging. Now at 67, she has increased the duration of her Indoor Rowing to one hour daily.

## 2. Rose- Displaced Fracture of the ankle

She came to see me some 6 years ago with this fracture of the ankle she suffered at the age of 76. You can see her pictures below.

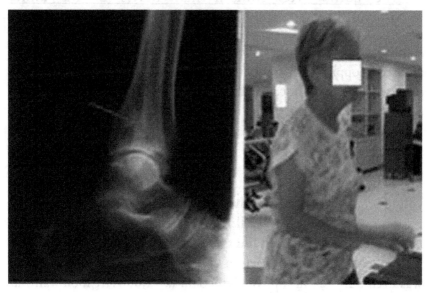

She was worried that she might not be able to run in a Veteran's competition 2 months later. When she saw a doctor, he remarked that at her age it was unlikely for her to recover to run again in competition. I rehabilitated her on the Indoor Rower, and 2 months later she took part in the Veteran's Athletic competition, and came back to show me three Gold medals she had won:

- 5,000m racewalk
- 200m sprint
- 100m sprint in 24 seconds

Just to show that it was no fluke, and that she had recovered completely, she broke the record the next year, and improved her 100m sprint in 23.4 seconds at the age of 77!

This again demonstrates the effects of exercise on Anti Aging, as conventional thinking would have labeled such a person *as over the hill as an athlete*. This is a remarkable recovery that has been documented by me.

## 3. The author KC himself had MRIs of his ankle diagnosing:

Achilles Tendinosis. Doctors and healthcare professionals had advised stopping all competitions or marathon running or leg squats, as these might cause the Achilles tendon to rupture one day. So the heavy weight training and marathon running were stopped, but high level competition at racewalking and Indoor Rowing were started seven years ago.

He is now a champion endurance Indoor Rower at 67, beating youngsters half his age, and has won many medals at racewalking (5km and 10km) that he still trains at without taking any of the medications and restricted lifestyle that the healthcare professionals recommend. This can be seen in Chapter 2 (Indoor Rowing). There was even a hill climb up Mt. Kinabalu (a 14,000+ ft mountain) at the age of 65, where in the space of three months, the time taken to climb the mountain from the base camp up to the 10,000 ft rest house improved from seven hours to three hours and forty-six minutes. All this has been documented on the Polar heart rate monitor, and the downloaded recording of both climbs is reproduced here below:

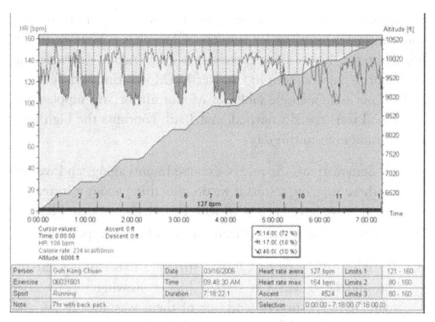

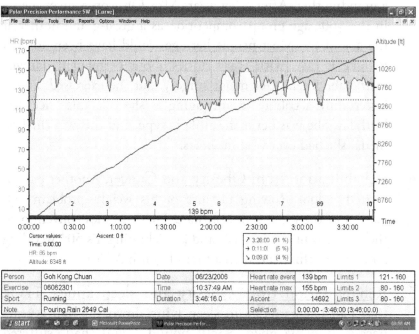

Family History of Diabetes, with a mother dying of its complications at the age of 58, and blood tests such as the Fasting Blood Sugar, HbA1c, and Oral Glucose Tolerance Test to diagnose pre Diabetes, or Impaired Glucose Tolerance, as it is medically termed. The conventional medical advice is to take Glucophage (Metformin) for life. However, I have been exercising on the Indoor Rower for up to 5 hours a day – as seen in Chapter 12 (Monitoring and Testing), and do not take a single tablet of Metformin or any supplement. The blood tests remain normal, and I still continue the high level competition even to this day.

All this demonstrates the role of exercise in anti aging, and we can achieve these amazing results if we do something about it instead of whining that we have been born with these bad genes, and have to live a sedentary life, watching from the armchair of a spectator

3.  Rehabilitation from Obgyn surgery. Two septuagenarians Flo and Mrs. M.L.Oh started Indoor Rowing shortly after major Obgyn surgery, and one of them was already 77, and a grandmother. After a few years Mrs. Oh won a silver medal in the >60s age group competition as a great-grandmother at the age of 79. Most people her age would have been advised to take it easy, with scary stories about permanent damage to the abdomen after major surgery, but she exercised, and it is certainly a tribute to anti aging as she celebrates her 82$^{nd}$ birthday. She was never the athletic type, and this was the first medal she had ever won in sports.

4.  Rehabilitation from Obesity and Cancer. Another patient started indoor Rowing because of his weight problem and Cancer of the kidney and prostate. He continues conventional therapy, and fits in exercise, and is celebrating his 50$^{th}$ wedding anniversary this year, with a tour of South Africa.

5.  Rehabilitation from Obesity and sleep apnea. Frank (60) had been unable to sleep lying down for many years because he weighed >330 pounds, and had suffered congestive cardiac failure, a stroke and Diabetes. He started rehabilitating especially with the indoor Rower, and lost 46 pounds in 5 months in spite of eating more than anybody

else (like a whole head of cabbage in one sitting). He almost lost both legs through infection, but rehabilitated so well that he could finally sleep flat on his back, went back to working night duty, and came to exercise on his superbike, as well as enjoying his favorite hobby of hunting wild game with powder rifles. This is his testimony:

Frank R. Ely Sr.
145 Cherry Street
Naugatuck CT 06770

To Whom It May Concern

When I first came to Wellness 2000 LLC Health Center I was suffering from the following:

- 6 years ago I had congestive heart failure
- A year later I had a stroke.
- Two years after the stroke I found I had diabetes
- A year after this my right leg became ulcerated, and I almost lost it
- A year later my left leg got ulcerated.
- I also had **sleep apnea** condition. I would sleep sitting up most of the night and also would only sleep one to one and a half hours. Then I would wake up and stay up for an hour.

I have been going to the Wellness 2000 Health Center for 5 months. I did weigh 334 pounds when I started. Now I weigh about 288 pounds. **I have lost 46 pounds in 5 months!** My legs have never felt so good. I also sleep three and a quarter to five and a half hours, and all of this is lying down and not sitting up sleeping. I also have about four times the energy I ever had before.

The Wellness 2000 Health Center has given me a second chance to live. My Doctor told me if I didn't do something real soon that I would have a very short life to live. I have tried dieting- never worked for me because I would go off it. I tried exercising by myself, but that didn't work either.

The Wellness 2000 Health Center made everything possible. Now I am enjoying my life, and also still going to Wellness 2000 Health Center. Dr. K.C. Goh is doing a wonderful job helping me regain my health back

*Frank R. Ely Sr.*
Signed.

*Franh R. Ely Sr*

3/26/2001

6. <u>Rehabilitation from hip replacement</u>. An octogenarian started on Indoor Rowing 1 month after she had a hip replacement because she had fractured her hip after a minor

fall on grass even though she had been on daily Fosamax for 3 years. She progressed on to independent walking, and improved tremendously in health.

7. Rehabilitation from multiple fractures. A diabetic septuagenarian came for rehabilitation because she had suffered a crush injury from a falling tree that had killed her husband out for his morning walk beside her. She had been desperate for help, and groaning in pain in spite of daily traditional exercise (Qigong). She started on Indoor Rowing, and is at it for more than an hour even now, after having been on it for the past 3 years. The pins and plates in her bones are permanent, and she manages with grafted skin and muscles. Pictures of her can be seen in Chapter 6, Fig 6.

8. Rehabilitation from severe headache.

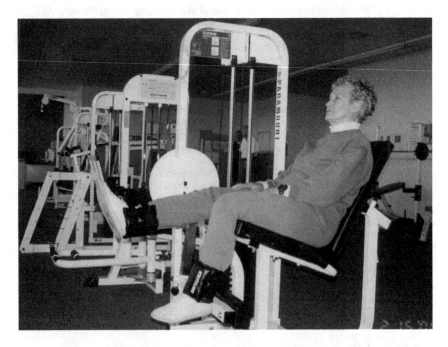

Abigail had been suffering from severe trigeminal neuralgia that has reduced her quality of life, and she wanted badly to resume her favorite pastime of dancing. When she first started she could hardly climb the stairs to her upstairs living room, and had to hold on to the banisters for aid. But after a few months of exercise, she could manage all these:

- Carry a 34 pound kayak out of her car and paddle in the lake
- Carry a tv set downstairs
- Jump on a trampoline the afternoon after slipping on ice
- Dance freely, holding on to weights.

That is precisely what we aim for- to return quality life to someone who thought she had lost it all when she grew older.

These are all examples of ordinary people who have not won Olympic medals, but chosen to continue exercising after rehabilitating from their injuries. That is the crux of the anti aging we seek to promote.

## Key Points

Many examples of how exercise plays a big role in anti aging to return quality of life to those who think they have lost it forever.

# 10
# Intensity of Exercise

Now that we have discussed the various modes of Exercise, we should know what intensity to exercise at. After all, this is like deciding on the dosage and frequency of taking medicine. You cannot simply take any medicine (even one carefully chosen and prescribed by the Doctor) at any dose and frequency you like; each medicine is different, and you do not want to suffer from over or under dosing yourself. You have to be true to yourself, and use the mode of monitoring that is most accurate and objective. For example, there is no use trusting a Pedometer that reads 4,000 steps one day and 14,000 the next, for exactly the same activity. It may make you feel good, but do you really benefit?

For those trying to lose weight, the concept of "Selective Substrate Utilization" needs to be explained. This simply means that

- At low to moderate intensity Exercise, the body selectively burns a higher percentage of Fats (even those stored as cellulite under the skin).

- At high intensity (of short duration), the body switches to Carbohydrate metabolism. So those who train at high intensity will lose more Carbohydrate instead of the Fat they want to lose (even as much as 98%).

- At high intensity of long duration (such as marathon racing), the body burns its own protein stores (from muscles), and you do lose more weight than from purely burning fat, but you will look haggard from the loss of muscles, and feel weakened.

- From this simple explanation, it is obvious that low intensity Exercise of Long Duration is the answer to the correct Intensity of Exercise.

Over-exercise at high intensity burns the body proteins as well as fat and Carbohydrate stores. The result is a cachexic looking athlete who looks like a starving refugee. (S)he is always prone to lethargy and illness such as Infectious Mononucleosis, and needs prolonged rest to get back into winning form. Very often the "Female athlete triad" strikes, and these female athletes suffer from Osteoporosis (as their estrogen hormones are not secreted), and they easily break their bones. Many of them also Diet, and Anorexia Nervosa or Bulimia may claim them as fatal victims. So let us be careful to find the correct intensity of exercise that allows us to reach our goals without leaving permanent damage on our health.

For the elderly, long slow distance (lsd) is the answer, the emphasis being on the word "slow". There is no perfect duration or intensity to recommend, as it depends on the individual, some gaining benefit from as little as 7 minutes three times per week, and some needing 30 minutes. Patience is a virtue here as always, and it is better to get results slowly than to suffer permanent damage from too high an intensity. These are the "kiasu" people, a type of behavior characteristic that literally means *"afraid to lose"*. They push themselves over the limit, and then become too scared to exercise anymore. It is better to read about this than to experience it yourself, and find that you cannot recover from it.

There was a martial arts instructor, "Big brother Weng" who was preparing for an exhibition. Every day he would set up this solid 5Kg weight, and push his palm against it. This went on for 3 months. Then on the day of the exhibition he just pushed a long nail into a piece of wood with his bare hands! From a simple action he had built up enough strength to perform a superhuman feat.

Some examples of the correct Intensity of Exercise are our cover girls:

- Nelly started with 30 minutes of Indoor Rowing, three times a week at a relatively fast pace of 3 minutes per 500 meters. Now she has slowed down to the reasonable pace of 3:30 per 500 m, and increased her duration of exercise to 45 minutes to row more comfortably, and she does so at the age of 88, with Osteoarthritis of both knees.

- Florence used to row at 2:50 per 500 meter pace for 30 minutes, but now, at 66, she has slowed down to 3:20 per 500 m pace, but lengthened the duration of exercise to 70 minutes and increased the frequency from three to six times a week .

- The author has shown improvement of 50% from a one month row of 1,006,000 meters when 60 to 1.49 million m at 66 (see the chart in Chapter 11). This only goes to show that we can improve even as we age, and this is the perfect mode of Exercise for anti aging. Let me reiterate- lsd- to increase the DURATION and FREQUENCY, but SLOW DOWN THE PACE, and burn more FAT Calories safely.

## Judging by Sweating

Does anyone sweat as much on other modes of regular exercise? There are many who feel they must exercise until they sweat, but do they really sweat this much? Until they really sweat, they do not feel the mode or intensity of exercise is good enough for them. They think they are always living in a dry temperate climate. They must experience living in a humid tropical region where you sweat even sitting down quietly or fidgeting at most. What is the use of trying to exercise until you sweat in an air conditioned room, when you are sweating sitting down quietly outside? Your heart rate may only be at its resting level of 72, but you are already sweating outside in the humid tropical region (with a measured humidity of 98%), whereas when you step into the air conditioned room with a humidity of around 60%, you may have to push your heart rate up to 100bpm, and yet not even raise a sweat. I experienced this in Texas where I stayed for 1 month, rowing >300,000 meters. How can you possibly judge your intensity of exercise by sweating alone? You need more objective feedback, such as looking into a heart rate monitor display, and you need consistency in exercise to reap health benefits.

Then again, there are those who try to strictly adhere to a "zone" they have calculated from a fixed percentage of the primitive formula of "220-age" that William Haskell came out with to predict the maximum heart rate. Many other formulae have come out, Leonard Kaminsky's "207-1/2 x age", or the ACSM "209-0.7 x age". Then Karvonen's formula is used to calculate this "zone.

I have a calculated "zone" above 130 beats per minute, but only exercise with a heart rate of 95-110 for around three hours a day, and an occasional 165 beats per minute once a fortnight. This will shock the serious exerciser who thinks he must maintain his heart rate within the calculated zone daily. We listen to our bodies, and use calculations only as a guide.

The calculations can be quite complicated, and serves only as a guide. There is no use strictly following this guide, and bandaging your knees to show the injuries sustained vainly trying to keep up to this "zone", or preening yourself with the false belief that *these zones are too easy to reach"*. Never feel that there *is no time*, and you have to rush through this boring task called "exercise" to *earn more money*. Many people feel they are too good for these calculated zones, and they disregard warnings from heart rate monitors telling them that they are exercising dangerously. So many exercisers have suffered Sudden Exercise Death (SED) or heart attacks leading to coma for not believing in their heart rate monitors. This warning is very timely for those who go to extremes trying to follow calculations.

High intensity exercise has caused arrhythmia in many of my fellow elderly athletes, and now they have to wear devices or undergo operations (such as radio-ablation) to treat this condition they have brought upon themselves through too much competition. The way to anti aging is to *Exercise for Health*, and not to keep on competing, for medals and the glory is only ephemeral, but we want to enjoy quality life for as long as we can.

## Key Points

- Analogy between intensity of exercise and dosage of medicine

- Selective substrate utilization for weight control

- Over exercise bad for anti aging.

- Patience and Long slow distance good for the elderly, illustrated with examples

- Dangers of high intensity exercise

- Don't use sweating to gauge your intensity of exercise

- Listen to your body, & heed objective warnings.

# 11
# Monitoring and Testing

Always measure and monitor exactly what you do. As in Medical Treatment, you first determine the type of medicine, so here we look for the best Mode of Exercise. To this end, the pace walked/run on the treadmill must be true, and there is no use fooling yourself about the pace when you hold on to the treadmill rails. The pace shown on the treadmill is not accurate anymore, neither are the Calories displayed when you hold on. These machines were calibrated with the subject walking/running without holding on to the rails, just as you never hold on to any support when you run/walk outside or climb a hill! Many a patient has suffered Sudden Exercise Death (SED) when running freely outdoors immediately after a stress test, where he had held on to the treadmill rails. He had been told that he had passed the stress test. If only he had taken the stress test without holding on to the rails, it would have given him a realistic evaluation of his fitness, and he would not have stressed himself to the level he thought he was capable of when he was tested earlier.

Next, we give the exact dose of the correct Medicine, and in this case we must give the best Intensity, and duration of Exercise. The advice given is to burn 300 Calories a day (Michael Pollock's recommendation for Cardiac Rehabilitation)[xi], or 2,000+ Calories a week (Paffenbarger's Yale Alumni study)[xii].

It is important to record your workouts immediately upon completion, and review them at least once a week, for only then can you objectively see any progress, and modify your workouts if you are not yet achieving your goals. It is no use blaming the Doctor for spending only a minute with you when you have the whole day to analyze your own progress. After all it is your own body, and you should take care of it yourself, instead of leaving it to someone else.

It is perfectly possible to do this monitoring, testing and recording, as that was how I looked after every patient in my Sports Medicine practice. Below are some examples of how to record and monitor your workouts.

## 1. Weight training workouts:

Every weight must be recorded, including the number of repetitions and sets, and the rest interval in between sets. You can do it yourself, or ask the personal trainer or person looking after you to do the recording if you find it too tedious to do so. I have seen an 80 year old meticulously record his training at every session, and he lived quality life to a ripe old age.

## 2. Isometric workouts

These are quite different from the common flexibility exercises, and many people think they are doing isometric exercises when they are actually only doing flexibility exercises. This is especially seen in those suffering from the common complaint of Cervical Spondylosis that gives s person that old and feeble appearance. They wring their necks up and down and all around in a vain attempt to reduce the pain and deformity that characterizes the condition. If only they had been properly guided to do isometric exercise correctly, they would not be wasting their time and become so dependent on their therapists. In the chapter on rehabilitation we have one example of a person who suffered from this very condition over 20 years ago, but has recovered to become a champion now.

The recording can be done in this way-

Write down how many seconds you hold on to each position, and the parts of the body where the isometric exercise is done. Most people only perform this exercise rarely, but give the impression that they do it daily, and that is the main reason why they do not get any results.

## 3. Flexibility exercises

There is a time to do these, and if properly done, they do prevent stiffness, injuries, and allow muscles to grow normally. We do not need mysterious names such as Pilates, Yoga, kick boxing, body toning and the like that are used commercially to attract members to these organized classes. Simple stretching is all that is needed even for elite athletic training. However, one can get along quite well without the need for formal stretching, and only the elite athlete or those suffering from injuries need practice them. In fact, overstretching before exercise, when the muscles are cold can lead to injuries. It is best to stretch when the muscles are warm.

You can easily record these flexibility exercises by simple ticking them off on you regular exercise chart.

## 4. Aerobic exercise

There are many tests used to monitor the progress of the patient:

- Kline/Porcari Walk test for the unfit. This is only 1 mile, and records the time taken to walk that 1 mile, including the heart rate achieved.

- UKK Walk Test for the normal person. Here the $VO_{2max}$ can be calculated from a complex formula for men and another for women. This can then be compared to the normal values for a person of the same age and gender, and the percentile ranking of the subject noted. One month after exercising, the $VO_{2max}$ is again measured, and the percentile ranking calculated to see the improvement. When such objective measurements are made, there is no guesswork in the assessment.

- Cooper's Aerobic Run- used by the athletic and Singapore Armed Forces trainees. You time your fastest run on a 2KM route.

- The Step Test- for patients testing out their fitness level. This is a recognized fitness test done at most wellness centers, where you step repeatedly up and down a 12" high bench for three minutes, and your heart rate is tested.

- The Rowing Step test- for those keen to test out their maximum heart rate. You monitor your heart rate as you row steadily for 2 minutes at increasing levels of difficulty, starting from 25 watts, and increasing each step by 25 watts. Some athletes can even go up to 600 watts.

Many other tests are available, but it is not the place of this book to go into so much detail.

## Resting Heart Rate

This is important to track because it tells you if there is any improvement in your fitness level. One may argue that this has no direct bearing on anti aging, but if you really want to prevent aging, you have to train yourself up to maintain your competitive edge.

Some of the training methods to really achieve a low heart resting heart rate will be described here:

- Interval training- where something like 14 two hundred m runs at 40 seconds are repeated, with a jog interval of 3 minutes in between.

- Jumping jacks, squat jumps and burpees that are used as weekly drills by athletes.

- Shuttle runs, where one repeatedly sprints a short distance of about 20 meters, and bends down to pick up bricks placed at these points.

Using some of these training methods, I managed to record these 2 heart rate tracings- the first showed a resting heart rate of 41 beats per minute, as against the normal of 72, and the trained athlete of around 40, while the second shows an actual training record .

The heart rate monitor has found its niche in those testing them out in the above tests, and gives an objective reading of the actual heart rate while exercising

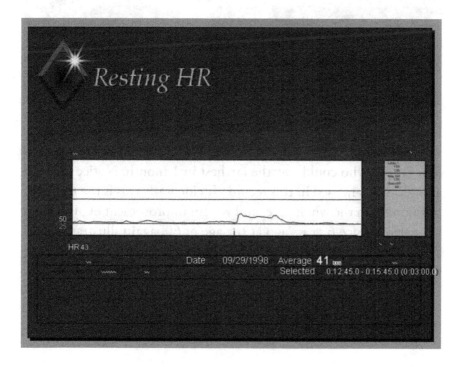

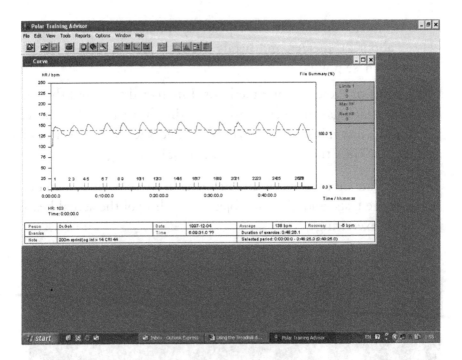

Here is a sample record taken by me during the 2007 NARC race where >3,000 rowers of all ages in the World competed against each other to see who could row the farthest in 1 month. Notice that not a single day is missed in this record. Incidentally this is the record of position #4 in the whole race, and was an improvement of 50% from the performance 6 years ago at the age of 60, again illustrating anti aging, as one would have expected a deterioration in performance with advancing age:

| NARC | MAR15 - APR 15, 2007 | | |
|---|---|---|---|
| Date | Daily Meters | Cal | Minutes |
| 15/3/2007 | 44232 | 2217 | 272 |
| 16/3/2007 | 45262 | 2285 | 276 |
| 17/3/2007 | 53189 | 2940 | 337 |
| 18/3/2007 | 44725 | 2243 | 312 |
| 19/3/2007 | 44416 | 2221 | 299 |
| 20/3/2007 | 52250 | 2618 | 333 |
| 21/3/2007 | 34105 | 1729 | 192 |
| 22/3/2007 | 22546 | 1152 | 134 |
| 23/3/2007 | 43965 | 2205 | 196 |
| 24/3/2007 | 43193 | 2164 | 269 |
| 25/3/2007 | 55785 | 2846 | 331 |
| 26/3/2007 | 51924 | 2469 | 300 |
| 27/3/2007 | 49894 | 2528 | 311 |
| 28/3/2007 | 46730 | 2264 | 279 |
| 29/3/2007 | 45198 | 2217 | 284 |
| 30/3/2007 | 44361 | 2291 | 295 |
| 31/3/2007 | 59603 | 3009 | 381 |
| 1/4/2007 | 25027 | 2199 | 127 |
| 2/4/2007 | 40331 | 2018 | 271 |
| 3/4/2007 | 43853 | 2194 | 278 |
| 4/4/2007 | 43159 | 2165 | 288 |
| 5/4/2007 | 36337 | 2807 | 242 |
| 6/4/2007 | 49208 | 2469 | 315 |
| 7/4/2007 | 48440 | 2407 | 245 |
| 8/4/2007 | 49929 | 2494 | 328 |
| 9/4/2007 | 58827 | 2971 | 360 |
| 10/4/2007 | 43677 | 2218 | 294 |
| 11/4/2007 | 53062 | 2671 | 337 |

| 12/4/2007 | 45705 | 2289 | 272 |
|---|---|---|---|
| 13/4/2007 | 43967 | 2201 | 284 |
| 14/4/2007 | 90531 | 4552 | 619 |
| 15/4/2007 | 38190 | 1944 | 268 |
| | 1,491,621.00 | 76,997.00 | 9,329.00 |
| | **46,613.16** | **2,406.16** | **291.53** |
| | **m/day** | **Cal/day** | **min./day** |

The first column shows date, recorded daily for a whole month (not even 1 day missed).

The 2nd column is the distance rowed, the 3rd is the daily Calories burnt, and the last column records the time spent exercising (in minutes). The figures in bold print are the daily averages. It is only when objective recording and monitoring are done that you can truthfully analyze what you have been doing. There is no use guessing and bluffing yourself, as the final result will show.

## Selective Substrate Utilization

This merely means that if you exercise at high intensity, the body burns mainly Carbohydrates, even as much as 98%, whereas when you exercise at low intensity, you burn mainly Fat, as much as 50%., but when you exercise at high intensity for a long time, as in marathon racing, you will burn up your protein stores for energy, and look haggard.

It was precisely using this concept of Selective Substrate Utilization that I managed to improve by 50% from the age of 60 to 66, improving from a distance of 1,006,000 meters rowed in 1 month to 1.49 million meters, even as I aged by six years, and have managed good weight control without looking haggard.

High intensity exercise also has the added danger of causing arrhythmia in many of my fellow elderly athletes, and now they have to wear devices to treat themselves for this condition they have brought upon themselves through indulging in too much competition. The way to anti aging is to exercise for health, and not to keep on competing, for medals and the glory is only ephemeral, whereas we want to enjoy quality life for as long as we can.

## Measuring Total Body Fat

Also keep track of your daily waist measurement (men, not to exceed 94 cm and women, not to exceed 80 cm), as this will reveal if your visceral fat is at a healthy level. In this way you may avoid the Metabolic Syndrome from developing (if you have a genetic tendency towards it)

- DEXA total body fat is the most accurate, and ranks #2 among all the methods. Here, you use the DEXA bone density machine to measure exactly how much body fat, lean muscle or bone you have in regions such as the trunk, limb and head. This has supplanted "Underwater Weighing" as the former Gold Standard for measuring Total Body Fat. There is also a "Bodypod" that uses air displacement instead of water.

- Anthropological methods, such as the Skin Caliper. Good equipment is necessary to do this, as well as a good operator. The Harpenden and Lange are the classic instruments, while the Lafayette is a newcomer. All others (like those used in many gyms are unreliable). It all depends on the number of sites and the formula used. 4 or even 7 sites may be used, and there are around 80 such formulae. Sometimes, Sum of Skinfold thickness (SSF) is used instead of conversion by these formulae, and this is the method of choice to monitor athletes.

- The popular Bioelectric Impedance Assay (BIA) where you pass a small electric current through the body to measure the resistance from the body fat ranks a lowly 6 among all these methods, but the results are very impressively printed out and presented.

71

## Measuring Endurance

- Stamina should also be measured, and in Cardiac Rehabilitation we are taught how to measure $VO_{2max}$. There is nothing to beat the Gold standard Gas Analysis method, where you have to wear a face mask, and measure the Oxygen consumed per minute of Exercise, with the value calculated to each Kg of your body weight. This is still practiced in a few good Cardiac Rehab centers, like the one run by the late Michael Pollock at the University of Florida Gainesville-he measured the $VO_{2max}$ at every Stress Test done.

- But most people just estimate the resting $VO_2$ as 3.5 ml of $O_2$ per min. per Kg body weight.

- Cycle ergometry, using the YMCA protocol is another classic method, and there are many books on Exercise testing and Exercise Physiology that go into detail about conducting this test.

- Rowing ergometry is a newer way of measuring $VO_{2max}$ This was the method used at the South African Congress of Sports Medicine a few years ago.

- Field methods are found in the ACSM "Guidelines to Exercise Testing", such as the Cooper's 12min Aerobic Run, the Step Test, the "Shuttle Run" or the Rockport Test 1 mile (of fast walking) or UKK 2KM Walk Test, (using various formulae) etc.

- There are so many tests, but the important thing is to test yourself out objectively, and record your results to see your progress.

- Medical screening, such as Blood Tests, Colonoscopy, various X-Rays and other procedures may pick out conditions early to stop the process of aging and insidious diseases that we are all prone to.

Very often, people think that they are exercising all the time, when they do it sporadically, and they only realize this when they record it daily. But most people are unwilling to do so because this will burst the balloon and deflate their ego. It is better to face reality and do something about it than to suffer from this false delusion and pronounce that their "constant" exercise is useless.

Anti aging results are best obtained with a combination of Lifestyle measures and Medical Screening. Monitoring and Testing give us an objective view of all this instead of leaving it to guesswork. It is worth taking the trouble to do all this monitoring and testing because there will be a noticeable improvement in your health and general wellness, and you would have truly made progress in anti aging.

My cover girls exemplify this fact by showing their progress from the front cover to the back chapter of the book- after a span of 10 years they have in fact increased their duration of exercise and lowered the intensity (objectively measured), and achieved their anti aging goals.

# Key Points

- Analogy between intensity of exercise and dosage of medicine
- Importance of recording different types of workouts such as weight training and isometric workouts, flexibility and aerobic exercise
- Tracking Resting Heart Rate
- Example shown for 1 month of rowing in competition
- Selective substrate utilization
- Measuring Total Body Fat and endurance
- Monitoring and testing give true picture of anti aging progress

# 12
# Dieting

No discussion on anti aging or weight control is complete without something said about the role of Dieting. This is the first thing that comes to mind, and Diet and Exercise are so closely interlinked that very often people seem to think that Diet "is the most important thing", and Exercise is forgotten "because it is too difficult to motivate yourself to do so". Most people believe that they must punish themselves in some way to achieve results ("No Pain No Gain") such as in weight control and anti aging, and the most popular method is Dieting.

Current theory is that *eating less helps to promote Longevity*. This, coupled with the study on the Japanese of Okinawa, Georgians and similar long lived old people is the current fashion, and like all fashionable trends, must stand the test of time to see if it holds true in the future. They certainly eat little, but they do exercise a lot. Let us take a look at the animal kingdom where we see that the fattest animals seem to have the longest life spans-namely the elephants. So is it because they are vegetarians like the turtle or is it because they are fat that they live so long? This is food for thought, and seems to run counter to the argument that you must eat less to live long lives.

We will not look at these theories, as they are discussed in many other books. We only want to spend time on practical measures that we can all implement immediately. We eat too much, but eating too little also leads to malnutrition, and leaves us with too little energy to exercise. The ideal balance is to *"Eat to Live"*, and only enough to provide us with the energy to exercise and not look malnourished.

First of all, let us look at the Vegetarian diet, as many people think that that is the healthiest way to achieve results. However, many vegetarians also suffer from heart problems and have to undergo Heart Bypass Surgery or Stents.

The elephant, the hippopotamus and the cow are the best examples of vegetarians in the Animal Kingdom, but see how big they are. The Horse- also a vegetarian, but the Clydesdale is a huge workhorse that eats the same hay as the racehorse. The only difference is that the racehorse trains very hard at racing every day. So, there you have the answer- is it the Dieting or the Exercise that is more important?

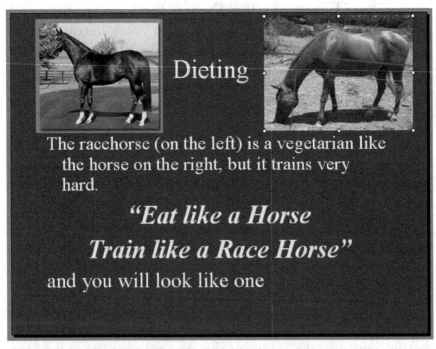

Dieting

The racehorse (on the left) is a vegetarian like the horse on the right, but it trains very hard.

*"Eat like a Horse*
*Train like a Race Horse"*
and you will look like one

Many diets have come and gone, as fashion dictates, but the Obesity problem is getting worse. So, do they ever work? It may sound hard to get started on exercise, but once you get used to it, and with the mode of exercise that best suits you, it will turn out to be quite easy, and only needs words of encouragement and some incentive such as small rewards or minor competitions where you win often to fuel your competitive spirit. You will enjoy it, and not need to punish yourself with a Diet that you will only take up for a short time and can't wait to get back to your old habits again.

Another point about Dieting is the misconception that it is useless to exercise because all those Calories burnt in 15 min. will be easily replaced by eating 1 apple. To these skeptics, we can only tell them to look at the end result:

Those who Diet always end up with a weight problem, but those who exercise never seem to worry about what they eat, and yet they have very good weight control. The explanation below should clear it up. Just look at the Resting Metabolic Rate. This plays the biggest part in weight control, and if we can reset it to burn Calories furiously while we are at rest, then we would have won the battle in Weight Control. We must always remember that when we diet, the body interprets this as starvation, and resets the Resting Metabolic Rate down so that we have to exercise furiously just to keep pace with this downward resetting, and it is a very tough battle to do so.

The following reference is taken from my attendance at the American Society for Clinical Nutrition (ASCN) in May 2003, held in San Francisco, and mainly from the paper presented by E. Saltzman and R.Roubenoff on OBESITY

While it is true that **Total Intake – Total Energy Expenditure = Excess Energy (stored as Fat)**

The Total Energy Expenditure (TEE) is a complex amount, and not just equal to the Exercise.

It also depends on the Resting Energy Expenditure (REE) that can account for up to 70% of the TEE[xiii].

If we Diet, the REE goes down, and it is too complicated to measure this in a proper metabolic chamber, while a calculation is too rough to give us a realistic figure.

Total Energy Expenditure goes by the formula:

TEE = REE (60-70%) + TEF (10%) + EEA (15-50%)

Where:

TEE = Total Energy Expenditure

REE = Resting Energy Expenditure

TEF = Thermogenic Effect of Food (the energy expended to absorb the food we eat)

EEA = Energy Expenditure of Exercise.

In a nutshell, when we Diet, the REE goes down, and we also do not have the energy to exercise, as our whole body shakes from the hunger and hypoglycemia.

So when 2 factors on the Right side of the equation go down while the TEF remains more or less constant at 10%, the TEE naturally goes down.

Look again at the first formula:

Total Intake – Total Energy Expenditure = Excess Energy (stored as Fat)

What happens is that there are now 2 negatives, so that we actually have more Excess Energy stored as Fat.

I want to stress the importance of the Resting Energy Expenditure (REE), also commonly called the Resting Metabolic Rate. This is always depressed in DIETING, and upsets the Energy equation by a large amount because it can account for up to 70% of the Total Energy Expenditure (TEE). So if we diet, we have to exercise even harder to bring the left side of the equation (TEE) just back to normal.

We often hear dieters tell us that they only have to look at food, and yet they gain weight. They never record what they eat, and we often see them gorging on their so-called low carbohydrate vegetarian diet. WHEN WE DIET, WE SLOW DOWN OUR RESTING METABOLIC RATE, AND MAY ACTUALLY GAIN MORE WEIGHT, as the body sees this as starvation, and stores every little bit we eat. The answer lies in Exercise, as this raises the REE and also the EEA.

When you lose a lot of weight, it is because you have lost muscle, as this sinks in water, while fat floats in it. Look at all the marathon runners and endurance athletes, and you will see that they look emaciated. The ideal situation is to lose fat, but gain muscle to look and feel strong and healthy. The elderly have that lean and hungry look called Sarcopenia, or loss of protein and muscle. In anti aging, we want a healthy person, and not one looking emaciated and feeling weak and faint all the time.

The next concept may sound contrary to what most people have in mind, but think about it:

> We should consider exercise as a reward rather than the punishment it has always been portrayed as, such as two rounds of the field when you are good (not when you are naughty), instead of giving out food (or sweets) to the growing kid, This idea becomes imprinted into the mind forever, and exercise has no chance when we try to introduce it for health or longevity later on in life. Who wants to take up a punishment rather than a reward, and indeed we need to be rewarded when we go on a cruise later on in life, and want to enjoy all the good food. When I went on two seven-day cruises, I managed to walk fourteen rounds of the deck (5 rounds equals 1 mile) every morning, when other passengers were sleeping. But I managed to enjoy all the best steaks and wines without any guilt.

Tasty food always limits your intake, for your taste buds have become satiated. Taste is a subjective sensation, and it takes someone from another culture to see how much people eat just to satisfy themselves. If only the food had been tastier, they would have stopped eating so much, and been satisfied with smaller portions. Satiety should be dictated by taste, but somehow this has been distorted to bulk, and most people eat until they are full to capacity. So let us not confuse taste with bulk.

Act instead of just talking about eating bad food and not exercising. If only more attention had been paid to action instead of talk, more would have been achieved. The focus has always been on eating, and this strategy has failed. Now it is time to shift the focus on to exercise.

It is not good for the elderly to Diet because of the danger of Sarcopenia (loss of muscle and protein) that makes them look so haggard. Malnutrition is also a problem many elderly suffer from. Actually the protein needs for the elderly are higher than for those below the age of 65, and the figure has been given that we need 80 Gm of protein a day when we are young, but as we grow old, we need>100Gm. of protein per Kg body weight[xiv]. This is to make up for the poorer absorption as well as the loss of muscle. But of course, the kidneys must be functioning well to excrete all this protein. But do people routinely test their kidney function? No. They only talk about it, and sound very clever at after dinner conversations, but they do not achieve what they set out do.

There are a few examples of the elderly who have retained their muscle definition with weight training, but these are the exception rather than the rule. In fact, too much weight training raises the threat of increasing the Blood Pressure during exercise that may cause heart problems or rupture of the arterial wall (that is by now inelastic) to cause aneurysms. So we have to be prudent when lifting weights as we grow old, but the answer to weight control certainly does not lie in dieting; it lies in controlled exercise.

Some people may quote recent observations that those who eat less seem to live longer, and medical theories, experiments on laboratory animals, and data on isolated groups of people are used. But the fact remains that manipulation of the diet leads to a change of lifestyle and "suffering". We seek here to improve Quality of Life in our quest for anti aging.

## Key Points

- Do not forget exercise in Lifestyle management
- Be practical- do not theorize on anti aging, such as "Eat less to live longer"
- The unhealthy vegetarian
- Eat like a horse, train like a racehorse and you will look like one

- Diets come and go
- The Energy equation
- The importance of changing Resting Metabolic Rate
- Protein nutrition for the elderly

# 13
# Prevention is Better than Cure

This is not just a cliché, and we read about many who are cut down in the prime of their life through disease. If only we could prevent some of these diseases, we could extend the life span and quality of life of man.

Drug abuse comes foremost to mind, and it is indeed sad when we see so many celebrities cut down in the prime of their lives because they have turned to drugs to help them deal with their stressful high profile life. The most widely publicized example is the famous entertainer, Michael Jackson.

There are many diseases Preventive Medicine has helped control, and if we are aware of these modern medical advances, we will be able to enjoy the quality life we seek. The many advances in immunology and vaccination have brought up the herd immunity to protect us from polio, hepatitis, German measles, even cervical cancer and many other diseases. Advice on Lifestyle modification points the way to dealing with high Blood Pressure, Obesity, Diabetes and some cancers. There is an interesting article found in Medscape 2009 that highlights the importance of exercise in preventing heart attacks among those suffering from Diabetes. The reference is difficult to find, because these articles on the value of exercise remain eclipsed by the plethora of articles written against it because everybody wants the easy way out- to sit in front of the easy chair watching tv the whole day, and buying whatever the media promotes as good for the health. It concedes that while Diet has been emphasized all the time, the focus should shift to exercise, as we can only focus on one thing at a time.

We have brought up heart disease, and now there is talk of inflammation being the culprit, and not high blood cholesterol.

"A study in The New England Journal of Medicine showed that women with high levels of a blood test called C reactive protein (CRP) which measures inflammation are twice as likely as those with high cholesterol to die from heart attacks and strokes. The lowest risk for a heart attack was in women whose CRP was below one-half milligram per liter of blood. Those who had both high cholesterol and high CRP were at very high risk for heart attacks"[xv]. This is found in the two references, the New England Journal of Medicine 2002 and Circulation 2000. So now the culprit seems to be not only high blood cholesterol, but inflammation.

Fashions and ideas will change with time, while the generations involved will be under the influence of the trends current to their time. There is no harm in exercising, and little research has been paid to this non-paying field, but the benefits are proven. Even in the field of cardiac rehabilitation, papers have been written attesting to the value of exercise alone, compared to the formal cardiac rehabilitation that involves the disciplines of Medicine, Physical therapy and counseling[xvi]. In a study they concluded that *Multifactorial rehab is no better than exercise alone.*

Osteoporosis is another disease prematurely claiming the lives of those who grow old. Most people accept this infirmity, and some take medication vainly to avoid it, but still end up with fractured limbs. We have many success stories of those who have managed to avoid Osteoporosis through exercise alone, but these will remain anecdotal because it takes much funding and statistical study to get them accepted by Evidence Based Medicine.

## Some Medical Concepts

1 **Aging of the Immune System**. Nowadays we hear more and more of old people succumbing to minor infections they would have shrugged off when they were much younger, and terms like Methicillin Resistant Staph Aureus (MRSA)[xvii] frighten us from staying any longer in hospital than necessary. Another term, Hospital Acquired Pneumonia (HAP)[xviii] has come into the vocabulary of Chest Physicians, and that means infection by a lethal resistant organism picked up while in Hospital. These bacteriae have become resistant to the most recent antibiotics, and are floating around in hospitals.

It is much better to build up our own immune system through long mild exercise than depend on the latest antibiotics to fight off a stubborn infection, as more and more bugs become resistant to them. No man-made antibiotic can ever match the natural defenses we have been born with, and if we can stimulate the body to keep its immune system always primed, we can best fight off these infections. It is important to find the correct intensity of exercise, as mild to moderate intensity exercise builds up the immune system, while high intensity exercise breaks it down. We hear this so often when great athletes suffer from diseases that break their stranglehold as the champion in their field, such as Tennis, Golf or whatever sport they dominate. One of the common diseases is Infectious Mononucleosis that has cut short the careers of many famous Tennis players. Another is the female athlete triad, where the stress, dieting and intense training has cut down their natural secretion of estrogen and caused Osteoporosis, with stress fractures.

**Immunosenescence** (the aging of the Immune system) **and Adrenopause** (the imbalance of immunosuppression over immunoenhancement through the cessation of DHEAS over cortisol overproduction) is the topic of a lecture[xix], but if we can somehow slow it down we can achieve Quality Life as we age, for Longevity can be expressed by this equation:

$$L = GMC^2, \text{ where}$$

$$L = \text{Longevity}$$

$$G = \text{Genes}$$

$$M = \text{Milieu (environment)}$$

$$C = \text{Chance}$$

It has often been thought that longevity is something we are born with, i.e. it is purely Genetic. But is that really so? In this formula we see that so many other factors must also be considered. Is it only nature, and not nurture also that determines how long we live? Surely the environment we live in, and how we live matters. Then again, we may have been living right, and born with Longevity in our genes, but no one can predict a traffic accident or a robber (who kills for money), or anticipate some quirk of fate. That is why Chance is squared in this formula. Perhaps now we can better understand the many factors Longevity is dependent upon.

Immunosenescence simply means that our immune system becomes less effective as we age, and we become more prone to infections that always float around us. At the molecular level, this is a complex explanation, involving the various cells and secretions that make up the defense system of the body. Terms such as Natural Killer cells, interleukin, T and B lymphocytes are mentioned in this explanation, and it takes quite a lot of background knowledge to understand it, but basically, we become prone to more infections as we grow older, and it only makes common sense to try to stimulate our own body to keep up its natural defenses. This we can achieve through moderate exercise.

2. "**Alteration of Gene Expression**"[xx], where we may be born with very bad genes, but if we can stimulate the correct genes to overwhelm these bad genes, then we can lead a normal life without the dreaded diseases like the many cancers or even diabetes appearing. This may be the answer to all the problems that plague us, and much needs to be done to really study it. To most people, this is only a dream that can happen only in the distant future. This is indeed the Holy Grail

of Medicine, and much work is being done on it. One of the many papers is being described here:

A group of researchers in California has studied how to use Lifestyle Management alone to treat those suffering from Cancer of the Prostate, and their results have been very encouraging. They found that 48 genes were "up-regulated", and 453 "down regulated". This paper on their research can be found in the reference given at the beginning of this section in the previous paragraph.

The net result is that these lucky old people recovered from the dreaded Cancer of the Prostate that is almost sure to strike every male as he ages, and did not have to suffer from the bad side effects of conventional treatment such as surgical removal of the testes. If we can discover the right stimulus, then we can prevent these dreaded diseases from appearing, or treating them with Lifestyle modification, and live Quality Life as we grow old only in numbers. This study was actually conducted by a group of researchers in California, and published in the reference shown. It shows that we can treat Cancer of the prostate in elderly men by Lifestyle Change rather than the conventional Radiotherapy or Surgery recommended. A lot more work remains to be done before this method of treatment gets accepted by the Medical community as the standard treatment, but it points the way to avoidance of the dreaded complications of radiotherapy and the side effects from drug therapy in Cancer.

Exercise not only gives us a chance to achieve *Mens Sana in Corpore Sano* (A Sound Mind in a Sound Body), or *Anime Sana In Corpore Sano* (A Sound Spirit in a Sound Body). This is the acronym for the famous Japanese running shoe company ASICS. It confers upon us Quality Life as we age, and as clear a mind as we would love to have in old age- free from senility or Alzheimer's disease, and above all, free from the physical or pecuniary side effects of Drugs- the silent thief. How it does this is through the release of:-

## 3. eNOS (endometrial Nitric Oxide Synthase).

eNos release is the buzz word in medical circles, and this relates to the release of the gas, Nitric Oxide when you exercise. All the cells lining your blood vessels release this gas (from the shear stress of blood rushing through during exercise) that dilates the blood vessels to prevent heart attacks and strokes. The same chemical is released when people suffering from heart attacks put a tablet of GTN under their tongue. The nutrition to the brain is also improved, and senility and aging are delayed when this natural chemical is released into our bloodstream through exercise. .

This enzyme is released as blood rushes over the endothelial cells lining the blood vessels. It causes the vasodilator, Nitric Oxide to be released, thus dilating the blood vessels and improving nutrition to organs such as the Heart and Brain among other vital organs throughout the Body. When this happens, coronary blood vessels are not narrowed, so that heart attacks are less likely to happen. The nutrition to vital brain centers is improved, and senility, Parkinsonism and other degenerative diseases is delayed. So we do not suffer aging problems at an earlier age. Perhaps this may be the ultimate answer to anti aging, and we only have to discover the threshold intensity and duration of exercise that will confer us this benefit without us having to depend only on drugs to achieve temporary relief.

## 4.The HPA axis (the hypothalamic-pituitary adrenal axis)

This is an important feedback mechanism whereby the body keeps itself in balance (called homeostasis medically). When there is a deficiency of a certain hormone or secretion, the body tries to make up for it naturally. But man has interfered with this natural mechanism by artificially producing supplements that give immediate benefit to the person. This may seem miraculous to the patient, but in the long run, it prevents the body from producing these secretions normally, and ultimately it is bad for the patient. A case in point is the well known practice of giving steroids artificially. I think we are all aware of the dangers of taking too much of this artificial substance. Many drugs and supplements are also marketed to supposedly benefit the patient, but in the long run they suppress the natural capability of the body to produce these essential secretions, and we age too soon. Another well known product is HGH, the Human Growth Hormone, but this has spawned a big direct selling business, and is well accepted. It remains to be seen whether this will benefit us.

- Vaccination and Immunization

There is ongoing research into the development of vaccines to protect us from many diseases, as viruses such as those involved in Influenza Like illnesses (ILI) and the H1N1 virus constantly change. This concentrates on the "Adapative Immune response". While the other natural body defense- "the innate response" is neglected. It might be better to try to stimulate the latter so that we develop our own body defenses against the changing environment of infective mechanisms. The innate immune response is non-specific, and does not protect us against one single infective organism at a time. We keep on searching, but if we can find the correct exercise intensity to *stimulate the innate response*, then perhaps we may yet find they key to true Lifestyle Modification and WELLNESS in the natural way, without having to pay for expensive unnatural medications that our present generation is promoting.

This quotation from the US Department of Human Health Services (DHHS) 2009 report is quite apt: *Finally, if we did not have an overweight and obesity problem in our society, we would still need a physical activity recommendation to maintain health and prevent disease. That simple message is lost on many who focus solely on the role of physical activity in preventing overweight and obesity. Consequently, the level of physical activity needed to maintain health and prevent disease is the baseline for any physical activity recommendation for energy balance.*

Perhaps this chapter is best illustrated by what one old timer said when he was lying in the Hospital bed recovering from surgery that had detected cancer of the Colon, and was echoing this common saying-" One ounce of prevention is better than one ton of cure". It sums up the attitude of most people who realize only too late the truth of the saying, and that this is not a mere cliché.

# Key Points

- Aging of the Immune System
  - Methicillin Resistant Staphylococcus Aureus
  - Hospital Acquired Pneumonia
- Build up own immune system naturally
- $L = GMC^2$
- Alteration of gene expression
  - California research on Cancer of Prostate
- eNOS secretion allows ASICS- Anime Sana in Corpore Sano
  - increases nutrition to brain, and delays senility
- Suppression of the HPA (hypothalamic- pituitary-adrenal axis) axis
- DHHS endorses exercise to prevent aging of the immune system
- An ounce of prevention is better than a ton of cure

# 14
# Real Life Anti aging People

- The late Dr. Paul Spangler once held 54 Age group World records from short distance running to the marathon, and also at swimming and other disciplines. He ran many marathons, and only finally died at the ripe old age of 95 while training for another marathon. What better way to go is there than to leap from one foot on this Earth into the next realm in just one "small step for man"? He still improved from his 25 min. for 5K to sub 25 min. from the age of 81 until 83. A "google" search on the internet will ring up many articles on his life, one of which is this:

**Dr. Paul** E. **Spangler**, 95, Dies; Took Up Fitness Running at 67 ...

14 Apr 1994 ... **Dr. Spangler**, whose first marriage ended in divorce and whose second wife died several years ago, is survived by a son, **Paul** A. **Spangler**;

There should be no copyright issues because this can be found freely on the internet.

- Another notable senior is the UK retired consultant physician who wrote of his experience, He recounted how he retired at the age of 65 because of a wasted leg through a slipped disc compressing on his spinal cord. He took up Indoor Rowing, and improved so much that not only did his leg return to normal size and function, but he became the 81 year old World champion at Indoor Rowing, with a time of < 22 minutes for 5KM!

### Reader's Letters: Kenneth Citron

"I have led a busy life as a **consultant physician in London.** During most of this time I took no regular exercise. But on reaching middle age I became convinced that my sedentary lifestyle could be a health hazard. Medical studies had shown that regular exercise was effective in reducing the risks of coronary heart disease, high blood pressure, cancer, obesity, diabetes, and osteoporosis. Exercise is also an effective antidepressant. This evidence persuaded me to take up regular jogging. Unfortunately I was forced to stop after a few years because of a **slipped disk in my back with nerve compression, causing wasting and weakness in my left leg. I had become a victim of exercise.**

"About the time I retired aged 65, my son left his Concept 2 Indoor Rower with me in my home. I started rowing gently and was delighted to find that it resulted in great improvement

## RANKING RESULTS 2005
### Individual and Race Results | 5000m | Men's | All Weight Classes | Ages 80-99 | 2005 Season

| Place | Name | Age | City | State | Country | Distance | Time | Source |
|---|---|---|---|---|---|---|---|---|
| 1 | Kenneth Citron | 80 | Esher | | GBR | 5000 | 21:42.0 | IND |
| 2 📷✉ | Stewart Hopkins | 80 | Groveland | MA | USA | 5000 | 23:00.6 | RowPro |
| 3 ✉ | Jostein Vadla | 81 | LEWISTON | NY | USA | 5000 | 23:04.1 | IND |
| 4 ✉ | denis melody | 81 | LEEDS | | GBR | 5000 | 23:50.0 | IND |
| 5 ✉ | william halleck | 83 | newport | nh | USA | 5000 | 24:34.6 | IND |
| 6 📷 | Rollin Foster | 88 | Bethlehem | PA | USA | 5000 | 24:53.1 | IND |
| 7 | Charles Ford | 81 | Overland Park | KS | USA | 5000 | 27:05.0 | IND |

The front cover and the pictures below are perfect examples of people who practice anti aging purely through Exercise. They show Florence at 58, and Nelly at 78 on the front cover, and many years later, with Florence now at 66, and Nelly at 88 shown below. Both maintain their health purely through Exercise, and illustrate the practical aspects of what we have been writing about in this book on anti aging.

Florence had Achilles Tendinitis from her high jump and long jump participation during her school days, and was almost sidelined with a severe neck pain some 20 years ago, but exercise has cured her (even of high Blood Pressure), and she is now the defending champion in the >50 and >60 age group in Penang for the past 4 years (2003 to 2006) at Indoor Rowing. She also wins medals regularly at the 10KM Penang Starwalk.

Nelly has been suffering from Osteoarthritis of both knees for the past 20 years, but refuses the knee replacement surgery recommended by her Doctors. Instead, she finds relief in Indoor Rowing, and has now increased her duration of exercise from ½ an hour to 45min. Most of her contemporaries are now crippled, but she soldiers on, and finds it hard to convince them that Exercise is the Best Medicine.

Both of these ladies have increased their duration of exercise, and jet-set throughout the World while their contemporaries busy themselves waiting to see the Doctor frequently.

The final example is the author himself, who competes against those 1/2 his age at 68, and still beats them at endurance. It is one thing to be physically capable (coming from a family that has Diabetes, Osteoporosis, Asthma, skin allergies, gout, poor cholesterol), but it is a great blessing to be able to preserve an active, agile mind as we grow older only in years. Perhaps these 3 pictures will tell all, as in the old Chinese saying- "A Picture is Worth a Thousand Words":

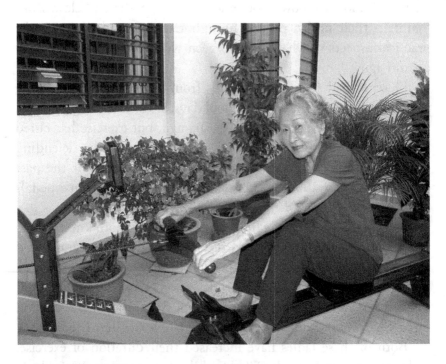

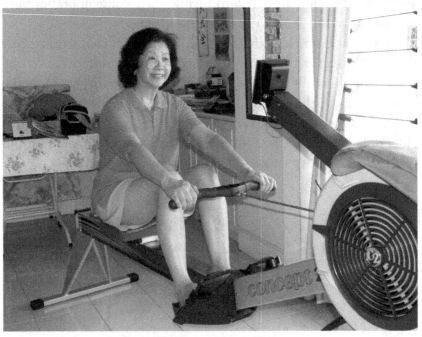

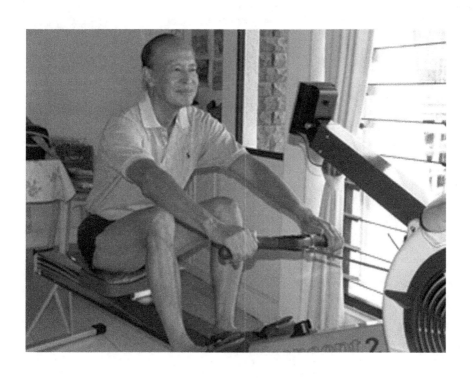

# Conclusion

We must be proactive about our health, and exercise is the way to go about it, instead of popping pills that are only man made. No matter how good the pills may seem, they all have side effects, and after a few years, many are withdrawn. Even the highly touted TZDs for Diabetes control are now the subject of controversy. The answer lies in our own body, and we must discover how to harness our own healing selves.

- Reverse our thinking so that exercise is regarded as the reward for being good, and food becomes the punishment instead of the other way around.

- We should monitor our exercise, screen ourselves for any illnesses that Preventive Medicine has controlled, and regularly test ourselves objectively to see if age or infirmity has slowed us down.

- Use well calibrated equipment, and accurately record the readouts such as pace, distance and Calories burnt carefully, without any assistance such as holding on to the equipment. This may be an effort initially, but nowadays we can do all this electronically and automatically with only one key stroke on the computer. Those who are extremely rich can hire someone to do all this recording and monitoring instead of putting all their trust in a Personal Trainer. Your health is your own responsibility, and important decisions such as this need your personal involvement. Ultimately the results will show, and constant exercise and review is necessary to fine-tune your frequency, intensity and duration of exercise that you will need to achieve long-lasting results.

We have gone through the various popular modes of exercise found in the gym and outside. This will give the reader an idea of what is available in the world of exercise, and he can find out about it without having to go through all of it himself. He can learn from the experience of others, and not have to suffer through trial and error.

We have also examined the concepts behind weight control and anti aging such as "Aging of the Immune system", "Alteration of gene expression" and eNOs. Some of this may be old hat, some is futuristic, but we can only achieve results if we work hard at it. The scope of anti aging is much wider than what we have covered, and we hope this book will help you in your quest for anti aging through exercise.

Exercise plays a great role in slowing down the aging process. It keeps the limbs and joints supple, the bones strong, and if we can compete against youngsters, then surely we have retained our youth. It also keeps our immune system primed, and prevents cardiovascular diseases and the degenerative diseases that contribute so much to the infirmities of old age. If the mind can benefit from this anti aging process, then surely we have discovered the "fountain of youth". If we keep up our exercise, we can enjoy quality life perhaps like the many examples we have shown here in this book. The remark is sometimes made that "Their biological clock has broken, and time seems to have stood still for them!"

There are so many benefits of exercise that stay hidden, awaiting medical research to uncover; and if we were to wait for these to be recommended by Evidence Based Medicine (in the many guidelines that restrict Medical Practice), we will all become mere statistics, and it will be too late to benefit us personally. Let us take the initiative,

and let commonsense and the experience of those who have succeeded before us guide us on the way to true Health and Wellness.
The final take-home message is:

As Nike says *"JUST DO IT"* and may I add, BE CONSISTENT.

You can always adjust your intensity of exercise and individualize it to suit you to achieve your goals, but record it and go over it often. It is worth this little investment in your health that will pay you great dividends as time takes its toll on your body.

All this is to inspire you to "ADD LIFE TO YOUR YEARS", and hopefully you will be proactive when you put this book down. When someone compliments you on looking much younger than your years (like my two cover girls), just quietly say "I ROW ON THE CONCEPT2 Indoor Rower".

# (Endnotes)

i    Indoor Rowing For Bone Health By Andrew Hamilton BSc Hons MRSC

ii   Indoor Rowing For Bone Health by Andrew Hamilton BSc Hons MRSC

iii  "Talk, Sing. Gasp" as an Intensity Measure- DEVELOPING AND MANAGING CARDIAC REHABILITATION PROGRAMS—Linda Hall 1993 page 77

iv  Borg Rating of Perceived Exertion (RPE)- ACSM GUIDELINES FOR EXERCISE TESTNG AND PRESCRIPTION 4th Edition pp69,70

v   The Multi System Effect of Exercise Training/Nutritional Support During Prolonged Bed Rest Deconditioning:An Integrated Approach to Countermeasure Development Heart Lungs, Muscle and Bone by J Hastings, P Snell, B. D. Levine et al.- Department of Internal Medicine, University of Texas, Southwestern Medical Center, Dallas, Tx

vi  Smart exercise: burning fat, getting fit by Covert Bailey

vii  LORE OF RUNNING by Tim Noakes, MD, DSc

viii Arterial blood pressure response to heavy resistance exercise by J. D. MacDougall, D. Tuxen, D. G. Sale, J. R. Moroz and J. R. Sutton (Journal of Applied Physiology, Vol 58, Issue 3 785-790)

ix The New York Times July 24th, 2005..

x Effects of pedal rate on respiratory responses to incremental bicycle work. By N Takano J Physiol. 1988 February; 396: 389–397.

xi Heart Disease and Rehabilitation by Michael L. Pollock Donald H. Schmidt 3rd edition page 247 Fig 1-3

xii Epidemiology, Behavior Change, and Intervention in Chronic Disease by Linda Hall c. Curt Meyer Page 10-, Figs. 2-5

xiii Obesity and Related Health Risks by Ronenn Roubenoff, MD, MHS, MIllennium Pharmaceuticals, Inc., Cambridge, MA during the ACSM and ASCN conference Tuesday May 27, 2003 San Francisco.

xiv Optimal protein intake in the elderly by Wolfe RR, Miller SL, Miller KB in Clin Nutr. 2008 Oct;27(5):675-84. Epub 2008 Sep 25.

xv 1) NEJM, November 2002
2) Circulation 2000; 102: 2329-2346

xvi Exercise-Bases Rehabilitation for Patients with Coronary Heart Disease:Systematic Review and Meta-analysis of Randomized Control Trials Am. J. of Med. 2004;116:682-693 by Rod S. Taylor, Allan Brown et al.

xvii Mayo clinic from a google search on the Web

xviii Harrison's Principles of Internal Medicine 16th Edition, The McGraw-Hill Companies, ISBN 0-07-140235-7(from a google search on the Web)

Printed in the United States
by Baker & Taylor Publisher Services

Printed in the United States
by Baker & Taylor Publisher Services